# Herbal Home remedy: A Beginner's Guide to Natural Remedies

## Step-by-Step Recipes for Natural Wellness and Everyday Healing

Rebecca Peters

# Table of contents

# INTRODUCTION TO HERBAL REMEDIES

## The History and Philosophy of Herbal Medicine

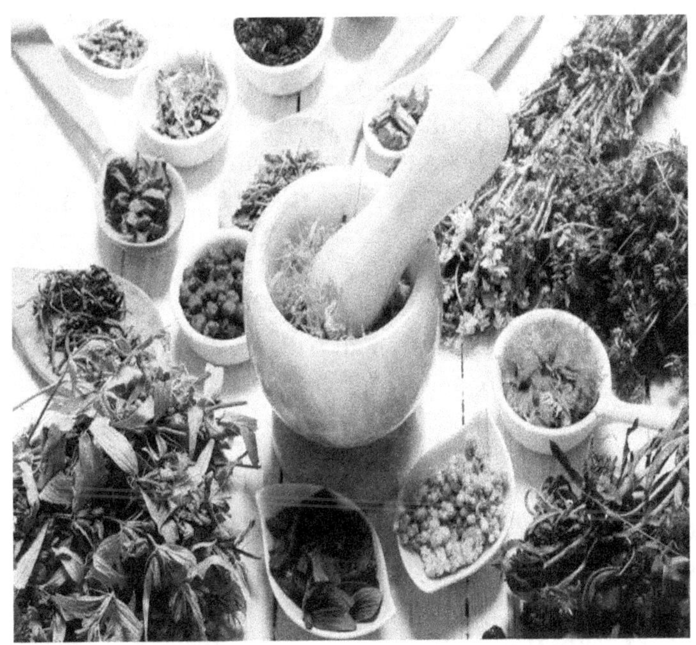

### Overview of Herbal Treatments

Herbal medicine's philosophy and history

Phytotherapy, another name for herbal medicine, is among the oldest medical practices in human history. For thousands of years, it has served as the foundation of traditional medical systems all across the globe. Plants have long been used for medicinal reasons; in fact, many ancient civilizations owe much of their cultural heritage to this practice.

## Ancient Origins

Herbal medicine has its origins in prehistoric times when primitive people depended on the natural world for both treatment and nutrition. It is possible that medicinal herbs were used 60,000 years ago, during the Paleolithic period, based on archaeological data. The use of plants for ceremonial, spiritual, and medical reasons has been described in ancient books and scriptures from civilizations such as the Sumerian, Egyptian, Chinese, and Indian ones.

## Philosophical Foundations

The concepts of harmony and balance are fundamental to the philosophy of herbal therapy. It is predicated on the idea that balance exists both within the body and between it and its surroundings in a state of health. Herbs are seen as holistic beings having energy aspects that may affect the mind, body, and spirit, rather than merely as physical objects with chemical properties.

## Conventional Systems

Numerous conventional medical systems, including Western herbalism, Traditional Chinese Medicine (TCM), and Ayurveda, have developed intricate beliefs and methods about the use of therapeutic plants. Herbs are categorized by Ayurveda, for instance, based on their energetic properties and how they affect the body's doshas (vital energies).

Conversely, TCM integrates herbs into a more comprehensive system that also includes exercise, food, and acupuncture.

## The Rebirth of Herbal Medicine

As individuals look for natural and holistic approaches to health, interest in herbal medicines has witnessed a rebirth in the contemporary period. An increasing amount of scientific study is supporting the medicinal benefits of many traditional plants, which is what is driving this renaissance. Herbal medicine provides a supplementary route to health and well-being by bridging the gap between traditional knowledge and modern science.

## The Herbalist's Function

Understanding the intricate connections that exist between various plants and the human body is a crucial skill for a herbalist. With this understanding, they design treatments that aid the body's own healing mechanisms. Herbal medicine is a patient-centered, individualized concept that often entails a thorough evaluation of a person's mental, emotional, and spiritual well-being.

Herbal medicine's philosophy and history serve as a constant reminder of our intimate relationship to nature. It inspires us to see health as a thriving condition of whole well-being rather than just the absence of sickness. We pay tribute to the historical customs that influenced our conception of health and the natural remedies that have improved our lives as we delve further into the complex field of plant-based healing.

This introduction lays the groundwork for readers to understand the rich historical and philosophical background that supports this age-old practice while delving further into the useful applications of herbal home medicines.

# Understanding the Basics: What Are Herbal Remedies?

Plant-based medicines known as herbal remedies are used to cure or prevent illnesses as well as to enhance overall health and wellbeing. The whole plant or certain plant parts, such as leaves, roots, flowers, or seeds, are used in herbal medicines, as opposed to pharmaceutical medications, which often contain isolated active components. This all-encompassing strategy is based on the idea that the intricate interactions among the plant's constituents are what give it its medicinal properties.

### The Fundamentals of Herbal Medicines

The idea that nature provides an abundance of plants with therapeutic qualities is at the foundation of herbal treatments. These treatments promote and strengthen the body's inherent healing abilities by interacting with its natural processes. They are applied in a number of ways, such as:

**Teas**: One of the easiest and most common methods to ingest medicinal plants is via herbal teas, which are made by steeping herbs in hot water.

**Tinctures**: These are small-dose concentrated herbal extracts prepared by soaking plants in vinegar or alcohol.

**Capsules & pills:** A handy method of consuming herbal medicine is to encapsulate or press ground herbs into pills.

**Topical Applications**: To cure skin diseases and reduce pain, external applications such as slaves, ointments, and oils infused with herbs are utilized.

## A Combination of Elements

Herbal medicines are prized for their ability to work in concert. The efficacy of the treatment may be increased and the likelihood of adverse effects decreased by combining different substances found in a single plant or in a mixture of plants. One of the main differences between herbal and conventional therapy is their synergy, since the latter often uses isolated, single substances.

## The Functions of Science and Tradition

Herbal medicine has a long history, with information that has been handed down through the years. Modern herbal therapy, however, also makes use of scientific studies to comprehend the pharmacological underpinnings of plant treatment. Herbal medicines are guaranteed to be both time-tested and scientifically proven thanks to this dual approach.

**Customisation and Wholeness**
Herbal treatments are often customized to each patient, taking into consideration their particular constitution, way of life, and medical requirements. The holistic approach of herbal medicine, which sees health as a balance of mental, emotional, and spiritual well-being, is reflected in this personalisation.

**Security and Performance**
Herbal medicines include certain dangers even though they are typically regarded as harmless. It's important to use them sensibly, to be aware of any drug interactions, and to know the appropriate amounts. Herbs' quality and purity are also essential to their effectiveness and safety.
An all-natural, comprehensive approach to healthcare is represented by herbal treatments. They provide a mild but efficient way to assist the body's natural healing processes and enhance general health. We become more and more aware of the vast realm of plant-based healing that is all around us as we investigate and comprehend the fundamentals of herbal medicines.

## Safety First: Precautions and Contraindications Herbal remedies

Safety should always be the first consideration while investigating the world of herbal home treatments. Herbs provide many health advantages, but they should be taken wisely and cautiously. This chapter will walk you through the crucial safety precautions to take to make sure your adventure into herbal treatments is safe and successful.

### Recognising Herbal Reactions

Prescription pharmaceuticals, over-the-counter medications, and other herbs may interact with plants. These interactions may occasionally result in negative responses while also increasing or decreasing the effects of the medications. Seeking advice from a healthcare professional is essential prior to using herbal therapies in addition to other medications.

### Acknowledging Purity and Quality

Herbal goods might differ widely in terms of quality and purity. The safety and effectiveness of the treatment might be impacted by variables such as the source, growing technique, and processing method. Select trustworthy businesses that provide open details about their sourcing and production procedures.

### Administration & Dosage

It's crucial to use herbal remedies at the recommended dose. An excessive amount might be hazardous, whereas a dose that is too low can be useless. Consistently adhere to the suggested doses found on product labels or those supplied by licensed herbalists.

### Restrictions

Pregnant or nursing women, as well as those with certain medical problems, shouldn't consume some plants. Certain medicines, for instance, may alter hormone levels or cause uterine contractions, which might be dangerous during pregnancy.

## Allergic Reactions and Side Effects

Recognise the possibility of allergic reactions and other consequences. To monitor your body's reaction, start with minimal dosages and stop using if you have any negative side effects. Rashes, respiratory problems, or gastrointestinal distress are examples of symptoms that need to be seen to a doctor right away.

## The Significance of Expert Advice

Using herbal medicines for self-diagnosis and self-treatment might be dangerous. Based on your medical history and present state of health, a qualified herbalist or healthcare professional may give tailored advice.

## Utilizing Herbal Remedies Sensibly

When administered properly, herbal treatments are a vital adjunct to medical therapy. To safely use the healing properties of herbal treatments, educate yourself, respect the plants, and pay attention to the knowledge of both conventional and contemporary medical practices.

In herbal medicine, safety is about making decisions that promote general health rather than merely avoiding injury. You may securely bring herbal medicines into your life as a healing and loving presence by following these warnings and contraindications.

# CHAPTER 1

# HERBAL ESSENTIALS FOR THE HOME

## Must-Have Herbs for the Beginner

Putting together a list of necessary plants is the first step in using herbal treatments. These basic herbs are adaptable, simple to use, and effective for many common health issues. This is a how-to for making your own herbal starting kit at home.

**The Beginner's Herbal Pantry: Chamomile (Matricaria )**

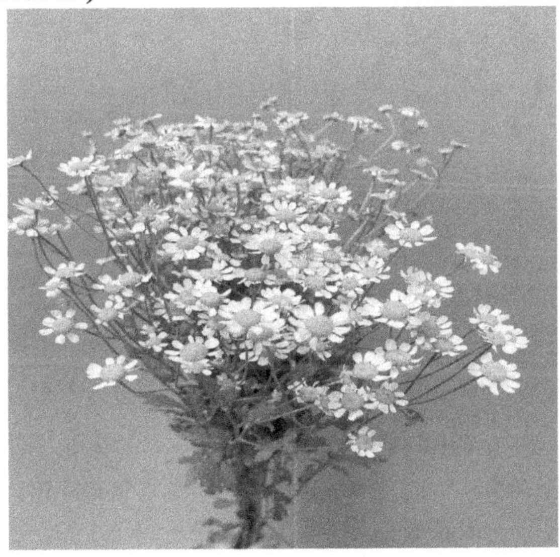

This herb assists with digestion, sleep, and relaxation. **Preparation**: Frequently added to teas or used as a component in topical treatments for rashes on the skin.

**Uses of peppermint (Mentha piperita)**: It has a cooling effect, eases headaches, and soothes stomach problems.

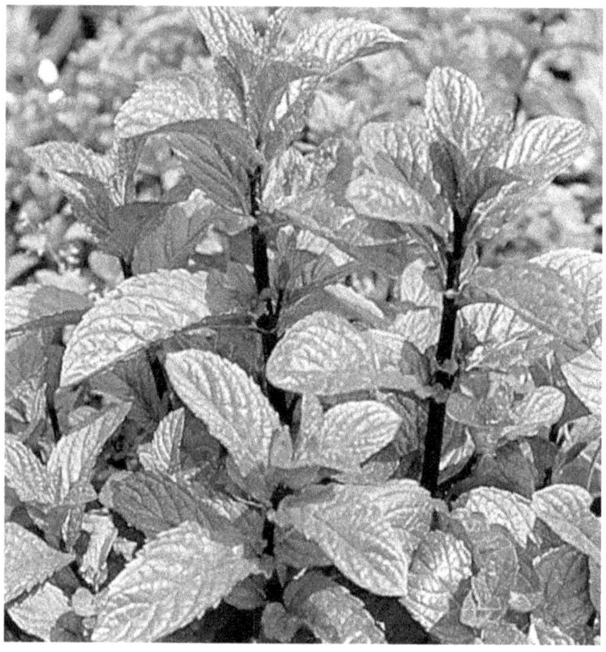

**Preparation:** Can be used in tinctures or made into a cool tea.

**Uses of lavender (Lavandula )** include lowering anxiety, enhancing the quality of sleep, and promoting healthy skin.

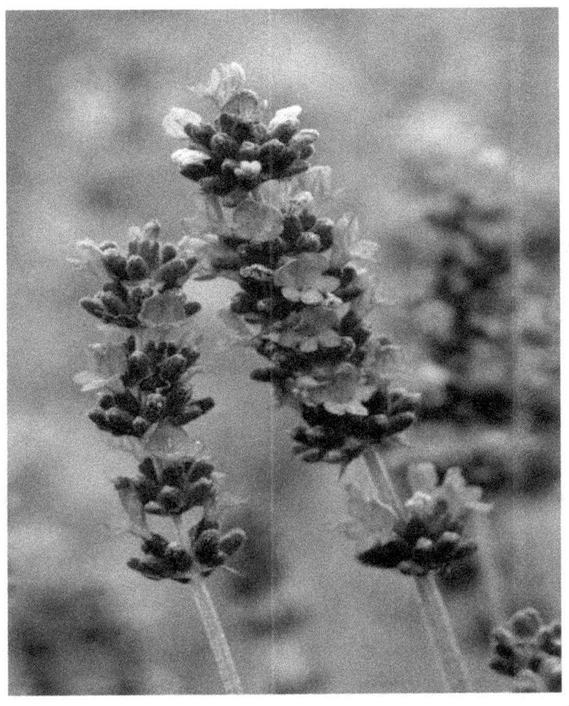

Prepare sachets, teas, and infused oils to have a relaxing effect.

**Uses of ginger (Zingiber ):** Reduces nausea, promotes healthy digestion, and reduces inflammation.

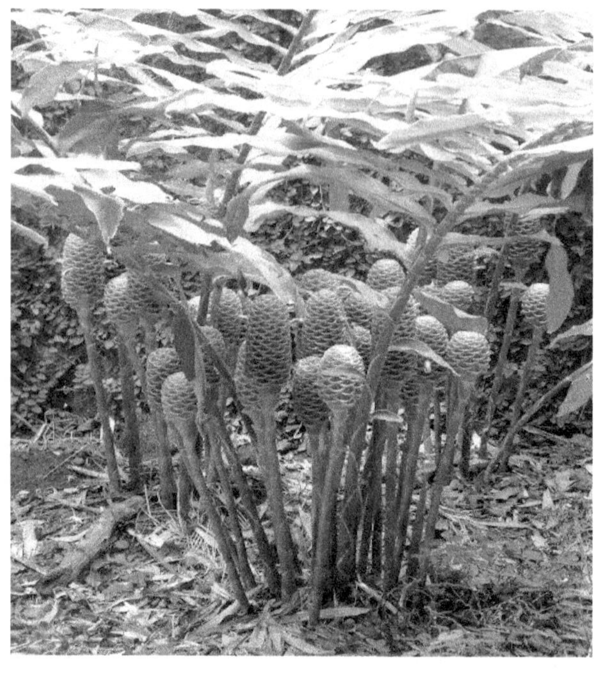

Prepared either fresh or dried for use in tinctures, teas, and recipes.

**Uses of echinacea (Echinacea spp.):** strengthens immunity; fights off colds and flu.

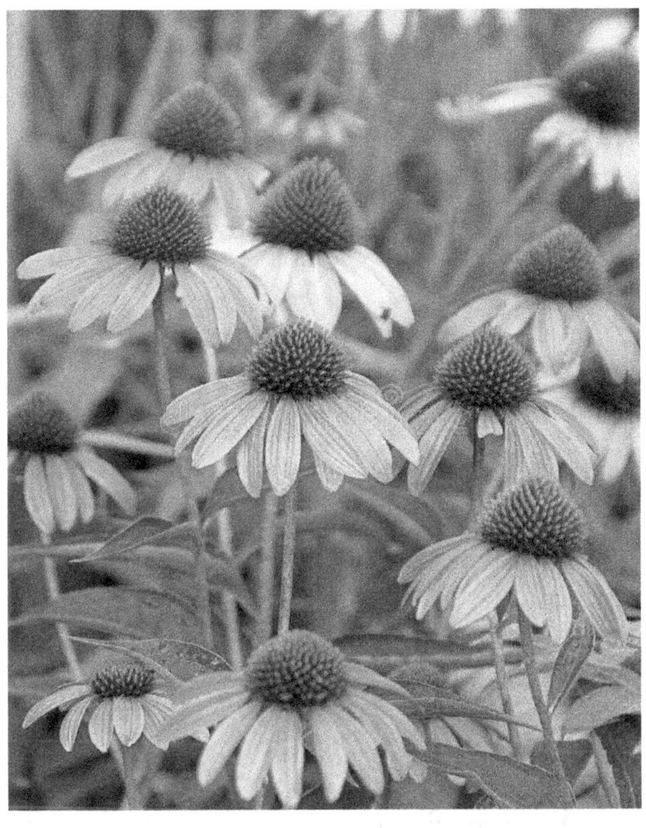

**Preparation**: Teas or tinctures, particularly when symptoms first appear.

Allium , or garlic, possesses antibacterial and cardiovascular health-promoting qualities.

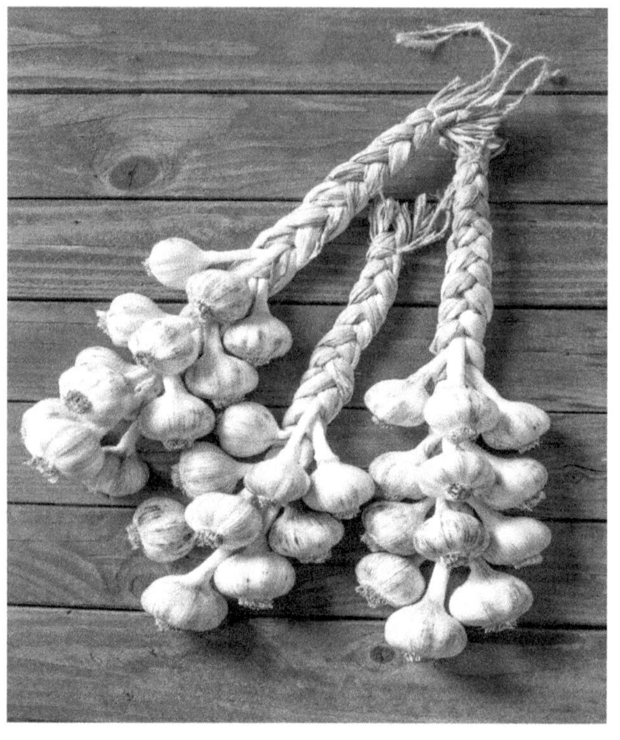

**Preparation**: For best results, use raw or as a supplement in cooking.

**Curcuma longa, or turmeric,** has strong anti-inflammatory and antioxidant properties.

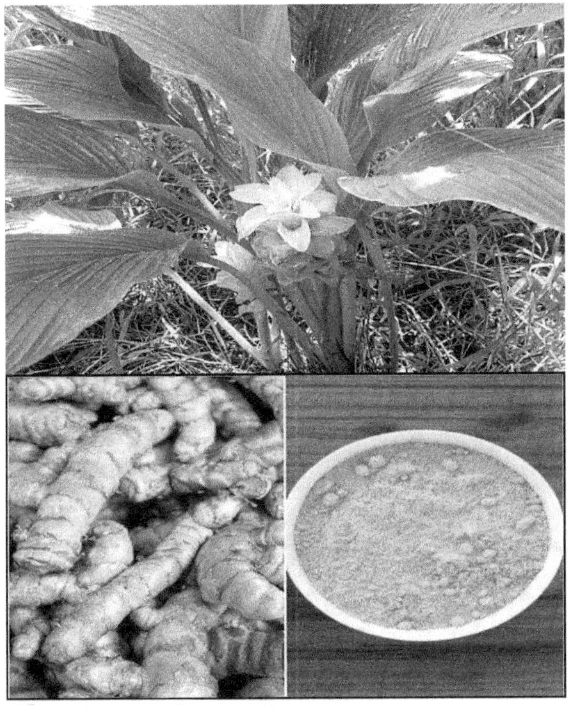

**Preparation**: May be brewed as a tea, added to food, or taken as a supplement.

Aloe Vera (Aloe   miller) uses: Promotes skin regeneration and soothes wounds and burns.

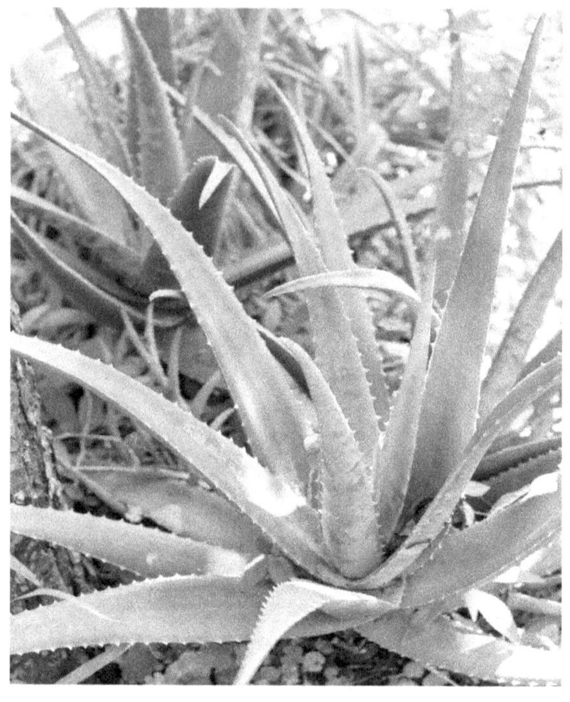

**Preparation**: Small doses of fresh gel applied topically or eaten.

**Uses for calendula (Calendula )**: Treats burns, rashes, and lesions on the skin.

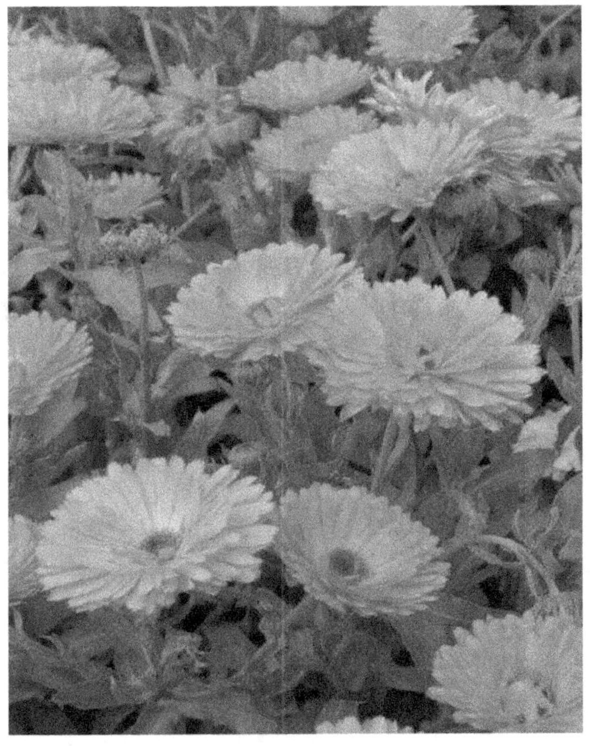

Oils, salves, or creams that have been infused for topical use are prepared.

Uses of lemon balm (Melissa officinalis) include stress relief, sleep aiding, and relief from gastrointestinal pain.

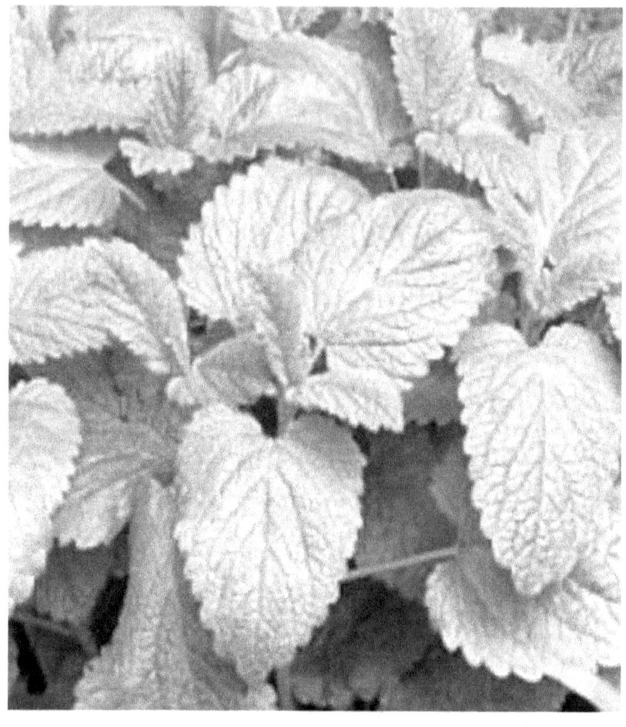

**Preparation**: For a calming effect, add teas, tinctures, or other ingredients to bathwater.

**Advice on Choosing and Storing Herbs** Quality Counts If at all possible, choose organic herbs to stay away from pollutants and pesticides.

**Complete Herbs vs. Readymades**: Making your own fresh concoctions is possible when you start with entire herbs.

**Storage**: To maintain their efficacy, store dried herbs in sealed containers in a cold, dark environment.

**Labeling**: To ensure freshness, always label your herbs with their name and the date.

The foundation of a natural medicine cabinet are these essential herbs for the novice. They may be used to make a range of therapies for common health issues and provide a gentle introduction to the world of herbal medicines. As your confidence in using herbs grows, you may add to your pantry and learn more about the wide field of botanical medicine.

This section offers a step-by-step guidance for those who are new to using herbal remedies, emphasizing essential plants that are simple to use and very effective. It highlights how crucial good quality and appropriate storage are to preserving the herbs' potency.

# Setting Up Your Herbal Pantry

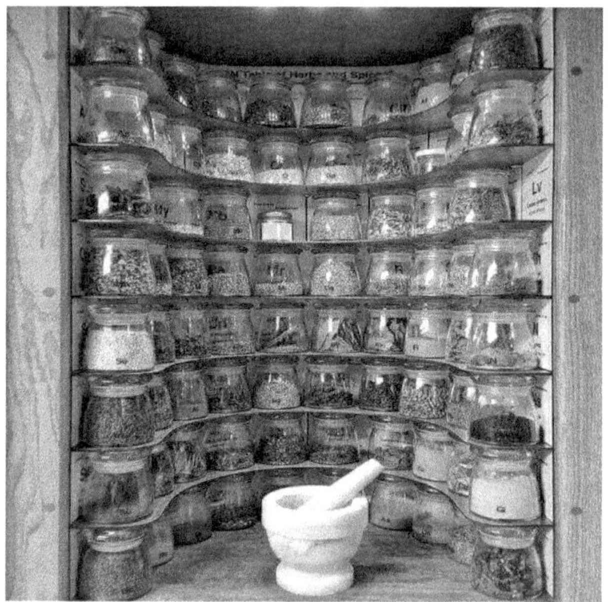

Establishing a herbal pantry is a thrilling first step towards living a more natural lifestyle. It is an area where nature, customs, and health come together to support overall wellbeing. You will be guided through the fundamentals of creating a useful and exciting herbal pantry in this section.

**Selecting the Appropriate Area**
You don't need a whole space for your herbal pantry; a shelf, cupboard, or even a part of your kitchen would do just fine. Picking a location that is cool, dry, and out of

direct sunlight is essential if you want to keep your plants potent.

**Essential Supplies and Herbs**
Start with the essentials and progressively expand your collection. The following products are essential for your first herbal pantry:

**Dried Herbs**: Common and adaptable include chamomile, peppermint, lavender, ginger, and turmeric.

**Carrier oils**: To make infused oils and salves, use almond, coconut, and olive oils.

**Alcohol**: For making tinctures, use high-proof alcohol.

**Jars and bottles**: A range of dimensions for the storage of oils, tinctures, and dry herbs.

**Markers & Labels:** Make sure your herbal remedies are properly dated and marked.

**Measurement instruments:** For accurate formulation, use spoons, cups, and scales.

**Cheesecloth and strainers**: Used to filter oils and tinctures.

To combine and ground herbs, use a mortar and pestle.

**Pantry Organisation**: Proper organization is essential. Sort your herbs by category, such as culinary, medicinal, or uses, or alphabetically. To keep your herbs, use airtight, transparent containers and mark them with the name and the date of storage.

### Sustaining Excellence

Keep an eye out for any indications of deterioration or spoiling in your supply. Herbs may last anywhere from one to three years on sale, depending on how they are prepared and kept. Herbs that have lost their flavor, color, or scent should be thrown away.

### Security and Availability

Keep kids and pets away from your herbal pantry. Make sure that the intended usage and relevant safety concerns for each remedy are properly labeled.

### Ongoing Education

As you add more herbs to your cabinet, keep learning about the characteristics and applications of each one. To expand your expertise, buy reputable reference books and think about going to seminars or classes.

More than simply a place to store things, your herbal pantry is an expression of your dedication to a natural, healthy lifestyle and a monument to the therapeutic value of nature. you  are making a significant step towards empowerment and self-reliance in your health journey by organizing and managing your herbal pantry.

# Tools of the Trade: Equipment for Making Remedies

Starting a herbal remedy preparation business needs the appropriate instruments in addition to expertise and plants. These are the unsung heroes of the process, they make it accurate, fun, and efficient. In this chapter, you will learn about the necessary tools that each aspiring herbalist needs to make their own cures at home.

**The Toolbox for Herbalists**
Making herbal medicines is an art as much as a science. You will need the following equipment to perform it properly:

The purpose of a mortar and pestle is to grind spices and herbs to unleash their whole power.

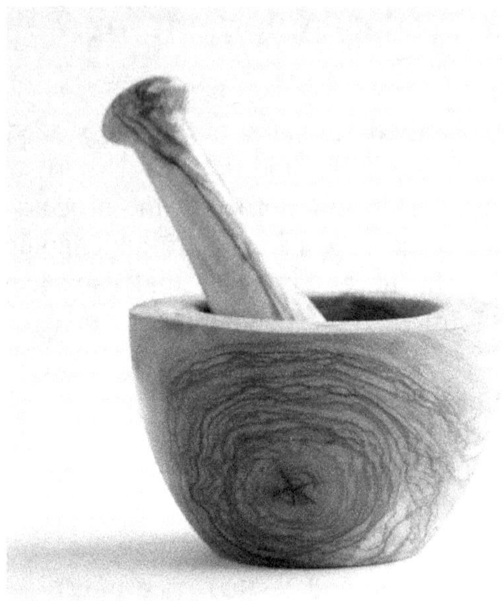

**Material**: For longevity and efficacy, porcelain or stone would be the best choice.

**Double Boiler**: To blend materials without burning them, heat them gently.

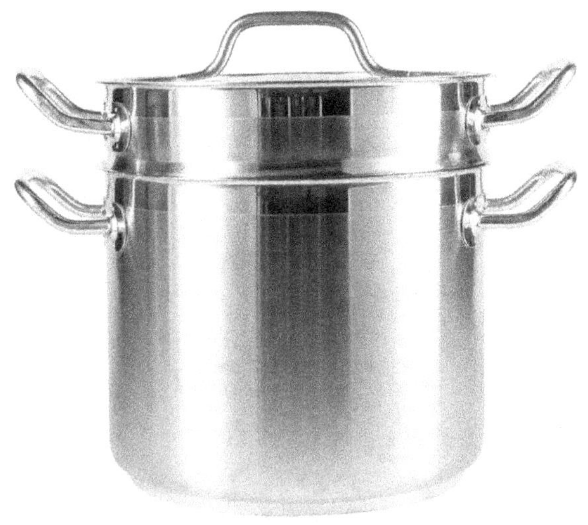

**Material**: Due to its even heat distribution and simplicity of cleaning, stainless steel is recommended.

**Cheesecloth** is used to strain herbs out of oils or tinctures so that the finished product is smooth.

**Quality**: Due to the natural fibers and purity of organic unbleached cotton, it is advised.

**The function of** funnels is to transfer liquids into bottles without spilling them.

**Variety**: A range of sizes to fit a variety of container apertures.

**Glass bottles and jars**
Storage of dried herbs, tinctures, oils, and syrups is the goal.

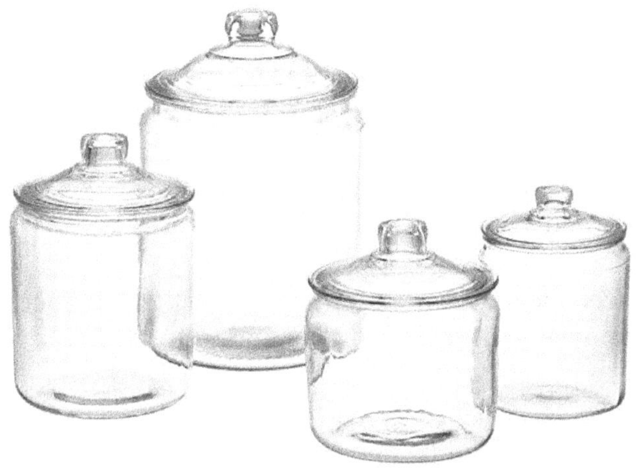

**Material**: To shield things from light and maintain their quality, dark glass works best.

The goal of the measuring tools is to guarantee precise ratios of solvents and herbs.

**Contains**: Precise measuring spoons, cups, and scales.

Labels and markers are used to identify contents and dates so that they can be tracked and used properly.

The finest labels and markers to resist handling and storage conditions are those that are waterproof.

**Carriers for Solvents and Oils**
Serving as the foundation for tinctures and infusions.

Examples include apple cider vinegar, high-proof alcohol, sweet almond oil, and olive oil.

The purpose of waxes and butters is to make creams, balms, and salves.

**Choice**: Candelilla wax for vegan substitutes or beeswax for conventional recipes.

The use of heat proof containers is for the safe mixing and pouring of hot components.

**Material**: Due to their heat resistance and simplicity of cleaning, stainless steel or glass are recommended.

**Organizing Your Work Area**
You should have a clutter-free, orderly, and distraction-free workstation. Make sure you have a comfortable workspace and that all of your equipment is easily accessible. Proper lighting and ventilation are crucial, particularly when handling volatile oils or alcohol.

**Updating Your Equipment**
If you look after your tools, they will look after you. After every use, give them a thorough cleaning, let them dry to avoid rust or mold, and keep them somewhere dry. Frequent maintenance will increase their longevity and

guarantee that they will be operational when you need them.

You are ready to start the fulfilling process of creating your own herbal treatments if you have the correct instruments. These instruments give the procedure a feeling of tradition and ties it to the herbalists who have gone before us, in addition to making it feasible. Accept these instruments of the art and let them direct you in creating treatments that nourish and heal.

# CHAPTER 2

# HERB PREPARATION BASICS

## How to Make Herbal Teas and Decoctions

Traditional techniques of extracting the medicinal qualities of plants include making herbal teas and decoctions.

**Herbal Teas: The Mild Brew**

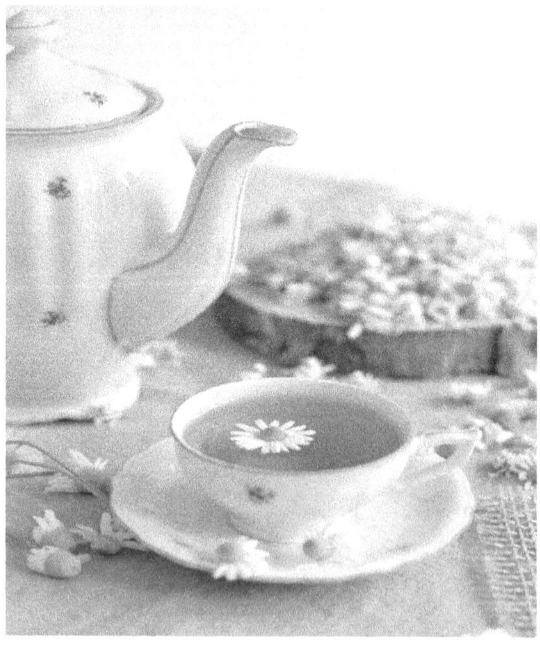

Herbal infusions, or teas, are an excellent way to draw out the subtle tastes and medicinal qualities of herbs, especially the aerial parts like leaves and blossoms.

**Ingredients**: Dried herbs, 1 to 3 tbsp
One cup of water that is boiling.

**Instructions**
1.Put the dry herbs straight into a cup or teapot, or filter them through a tea strainer.

2.Cover the herbs with boiling water, making sure they are completely immersed.

3.Put a cover on the container to stop volatile aromatic oils from escaping.

4.Depending on the kind of herb and desired strength, steep for 15 to 1 hour.

5.After the herbs have been strained, drink the tea, maybe adding some honey or lemon.

**Decoctions**: The In-Depth Extract
Decoctions are a great way to extract the strong ingredients from harder plant parts like seeds, bark, and roots.

**Components: One ounce of dehydrated herbs**
One quart of water.

**Instructions**: To enhance the surface area, 1.coarsely chop or ground the dry herbs.

2.Put the herbs in a saucepan and pour cold water over them.

3.Once the mixture reaches a simmer, cover the pan.

4.Simmer for 20 to 45 minutes, or until the desired level of concentration is reached.

5.Press the herbs to extract as much goodness as possible while you strain the liquid.

**Advice for the Best Extraction**
**Water Purity:** For optimal results, use filtered, fresh water.

**Freshness**: Make sure your herbs come from reliable sources and are in good condition.

**Heat Control**: Keep the mixture simmering slowly since too much heat might damage healthy ingredients.

**Patience**: To get the full range of benefits, let the tea or decoction soak for the whole amount of time.

**Storage**: To retain optimal efficacy, refrigerate any leftovers and eat within 48 hours.

Herbal infusions and teas are not just medicinal; they are rituals that re-establish our connection to the natural world and its restorative cycles. With the help of this book, you may create traditional and up-to-date herbal drinks that satisfy the senses and feed the body.

# Crafting Tinctures and Extracts

Strong herbal treatments that concentrate the essence of therapeutic herbs are found in tinctures and extracts.

### The Significance of Extracts and Tinctures
Herbal tinctures are preparations made with alcohol that extract and preserve the active ingredients in plants. For people who would rather not have alcohol, extracts may be produced using vinegar, glycerin, or alcohol.

### How to Choose Your Herbs
Choosing premium, organic herbs is the first step in making tinctures and extracts. Although appropriately dried herbs may still be utilized, fresh herbs are preferred. Make sure the plants are properly recognised and uncontaminated by pesticides and other substances.

### Selecting Your Menstrual Cycle
The menstrual cycle serves as the solvent for drawing out the therapeutic qualities of the herbs. High-proof alcohols, like brandy or vodka, are often used for tinctures because of their ability to effectively extract a variety of plant components and their ability to preserve food. Vinegar and glycerin are great alcohol substitutes.

**The Procedure for Extraction**
To improve extraction, prepare the herbs by chopping or grinding them to a finer texture.

**Maceration**: Put the herbs into a sanitized glass jar and cover them fully with the menstruum.

**Labeling and Sealing:** Write the date, the kind of menstruum, and the name of the herb on the jar's label and seal it firmly.

**Infusion Period**: Shake the jar every day and keep it in a dark, cold area. Usually, the infusion period lasts between four and six weeks.

**Straining**: Squeeze as much liquid out of the liquid by straining it through cheesecloth or fine mesh after the infusion time.

**Bottling**: Pour the strained tincture into storage-grade dark glass dropper vials.

**Usage & Dosage**
Tinctures are usually applied in tiny amounts, expressed in millimeters or drops. The potency of the plant and each person's demands will determine the dose. For individualized guidance, always begin with the lowest recommended dosage and speak with a healthcare professional.

**Shelf Life and Storage**

Keep your tinctures somewhere cold and dark. If maintained correctly, alcohol-based tinctures have an extended shelf life and may persist for many years. Extracts containing glycerin and vinegar should be utilized within a year due to their reduced shelf life.

Making your own tinctures and extracts is a fulfilling project that fosters a connection with the therapeutic potential of plants. You may make cures that are both individualized and effective with time, good technique, and thoughtful selection of herbs and menstruum. With the information in this chapter, you may go on a quest to master the craft of preparing tinctures and extracts, which is an invaluable ability for any herbalist.

# Creating Infused Oils and Salves

Learn the craft of making infused oils and salves to start your path towards natural healing and self-care.

**The Enchantment of Blended Oils**

The basis of many herbal treatments is infused oils, which provide the therapeutic qualities of plants in a convenient and adaptable form.

**Ingredients**: Your choice of dried herbs; carrier oil (jojoba, almond, or olive oil); directions:

**Herb Preparation**: To enhance the surface area of your dried herbs, finely chop or grind them.

**Oil Infusion**: Pack the herbs into a sanitized container and pour your preferred carrier oil over them.

**Warm Infusion**: After the oil has been infused for three to five days, filter it through cheesecloth or muslin to get rid of the herb particles.

You may either seal the jar and keep it in a warm, sunny window or in a water bath on low heat.

**Storage**: Keep the infused oil somewhere cold and dark. If kept correctly, it may survive up to a year.

You may use infused oils topically or use them as a foundation to make a range of herbal products, such as balms and salves.

**The Art of Making Herbal Salve**
Herbal salves are a great method to apply the benefits of herbs topically, offering the skin a healing and nourishing protective barrier.

**Components**: Herbal-infused oil
Beeswax or a substitute made of plants.

**Instructions**
Beeswax should be chopped or grated into tiny bits to ensure uniform melting.

**Combining the Ingredients**: Heat the infused oil slightly in a double boiler before adding the beeswax.

**Melting**: Until the beeswax is all melted, stir the mixture.

**Test for Consistency**: Cool the mixture after dipping a spoon into it. Beeswax may be added extra if it's too soft.

**Pouring**: Transfer the mixture into clean tins or jars after the required consistency is achieved.

**Cooling**: Before closing the jars, let the salve cool and harden.

Herbal salves are ideal for treating a variety of skin issues, such as small scrapes and bruises as well as dryness and irritation.

Making your own infused oils and salves is a potent way to connect with nature's healing gifts and an act of self-care. These are easy to create, yet they have a big impact and provide a little healing right at your fingertips.

You will be well on your way to creating popular herbal cures that are likely to sell out on Amazon and in homes worldwide if you follow the instructions provided in this chapter.

# The Art of Syrups, Pastes, and Poultices

**Making Infused Salves and Oils**

Learn the craft of making infused oils and salves to start your path towards natural healing and self-care. This chapter is meant to walk newcomers through the simple yet powerful procedure of using herbs' healing qualities in the convenience of their own homes.

**The Enchantment of Blended Oils**

The basis of many herbal treatments is infused oils, which provide the therapeutic qualities of plants in a convenient and adaptable form.

**Ingredients**: Your choice of dried herbs; carrier oil (jojoba, almond, or olive oil); directions:

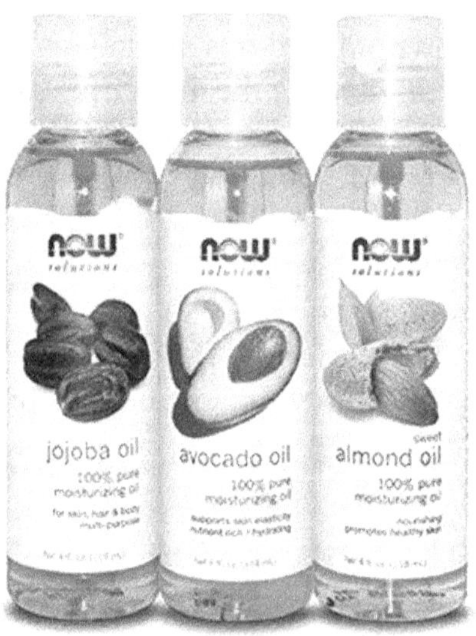

**Herb Preparation**: To enhance the surface area of your dried herbs, finely chop or grind them.

**Oil Infusion**: Pack the herbs into a sanitized container and pour your preferred carrier oil over them.

**Warm Infusion**: After the oil has been infused for three to five days, filter it through cheesecloth or muslin to get rid of the herb particles.

You may either seal the jar and keep it in a warm, sunny window or in a water bath on low heat.

**Storage**: Keep the infused oil somewhere cold and dark. If kept correctly, it may survive up to a year.

You may use infused oils topically or use them as a foundation to make a range of herbal products, such as balms and salves.

**The Art of Making Herbal Salve**
Herbal salves are a great method to apply the benefits of herbs topically, offering the skin a healing and nourishing protective barrier.

**Components: Herbal-infused oil**
Beeswax or a substitute made of plants

**Instructions**:

Beeswax should be chopped or grated into tiny bits to ensure uniform melting.

**Combining the Ingredients**: Heat the infused oil slightly in a double boiler before adding the beeswax.

**Melting:** Until the beeswax is all melted, stir the mixture.

**Test for Consistency**: Cool the mixture after dipping a spoon into it. Beeswax may be added extra if it's too soft.

**Pouring**: Transfer the mixture into clean tins or jars after the required consistency is achieved.

**Cooling**: Before closing the jars, let the salve cool and harden.

Herbal salves are ideal for treating a variety of skin issues, such as small scrapes and bruises as well as dryness and irritation.

Making your own infused oils and salves is a potent way to connect with nature's healing gifts and an act of self-care. These are easy to create, yet they have a big impact and provide a little healing right at your fingertips.

# CHAPTER 3

# REMEDIES FOR COMMON AILMENTS

## Herbal Solutions for Digestive Issues

Digestive problems are a typical worry that may have a big effect on life satisfaction. Thankfully, herbal medicines provide a safe and efficient means of promoting digestive health. In-depth, educational material that may help with the treatment of a variety of digestive disorders is provided to readers as this chapter explores the realm of herbal remedies for digestive problems.

### Comprehending Digestive Health
A complicated and essential component of the body, the digestive system has to be balanced and taken care of. Digestive problems may vary from sporadic pain to long-term illnesses, and they often indicate an imbalance that requires medical attention.

### Bitter Herbs: The Natural Aids for Digestion
For millennia, bitter herbs have been used to promote digestive secretions and aid in the digestive process. They have been shown to lessen indigestion, gas, and bloating as well as the signs of food allergies.

**Strongly bitter gentian (Gentiana lutea):** Encourages the formation of digestive juices.

**Taraxacum , or dandelion**, helps with a mild detoxification process and supports liver function.

**Cynara scolymus, or artichokes**, are good for the liver and help to increase bile flow.

**Herbs that Carve:** Calming the Gastrointestinal System.

**Herbs with carminative properties** are warming, aiding in full digestion, reducing gas and accelerating the process.

These herbs are very beneficial for calming the gastrointestinal system.

**Fennel (Foeniculum vulgare):** Promotes overall digestive comfort and relieves gas and cramps.

**Elettaria cardamomum, or cardamom**, is an aromatic spice that eases troubled stomachs and aids with digestion.

**Lemon balm (Melissa officinalis):** renowned for promoting mental and intestinal calmness.

**Herbal Treatments for Particular Digestive Issues**
Some herbs target particular digestive problems, relieving symptoms and encouraging recovery.

**Zingiber , or ginger,** is well known for its ability to calm the stomach and reduce nausea.

**Curcumin, found in turmeric** (Curcuma longa), has strong anti-inflammatory qualities that are advantageous for inflammation in the digestive system.

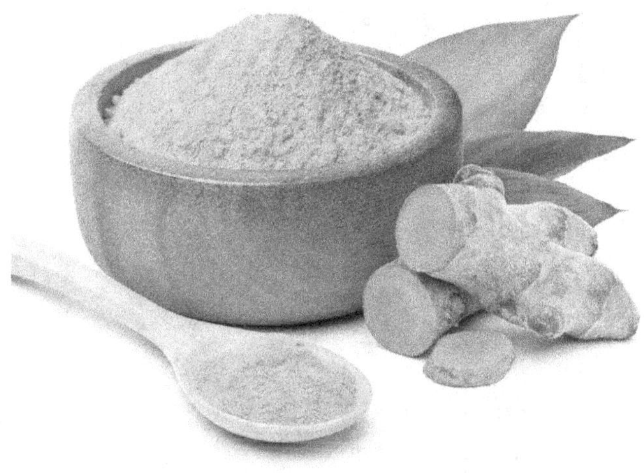

Milk thistle, or Silybum marianum, helps slow digestive tracts and supports liver function.

**Slippery Elm (Ulmus):** Reduces inflammation and acid reflux by creating a calming layer across the mucous membranes.

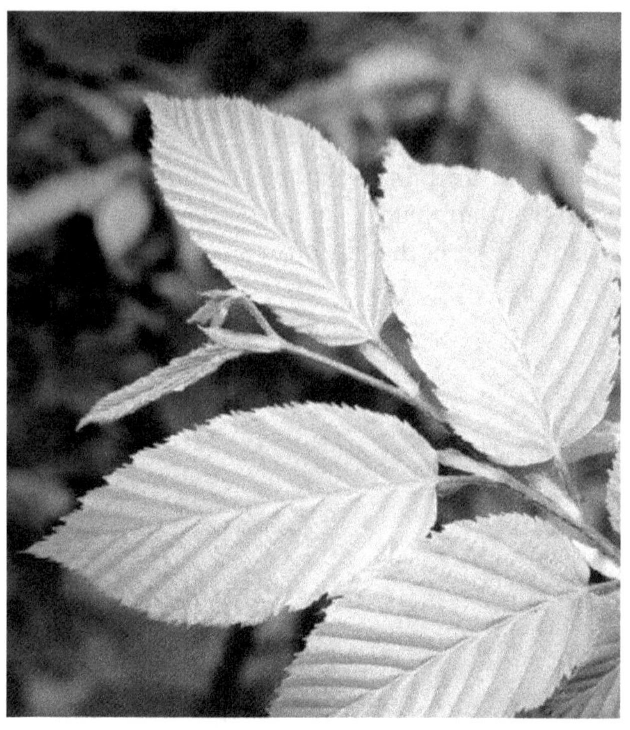

## Probiotics: Stabilizing the Microbiome

Probiotics are good bacteria that are essential for controlling digestion and preserving gut health. They may be given as supplements or found in fermented foods.

Taking care of digestive problems naturally and comprehensively is possible with herbal therapies. Through comprehension and use of the herbs covered in this chapter, people may enhance their general health and promote the health of their digestive systems. Never forget that you should always get medical advice before beginning any new therapy, particularly if you are on medication or have a pre-existing disease.

Beginners may easily understand the material provided, but experts in herbal medicines will find it interesting since it is given in a precise enough manner.

# Natural Remedies for Skin Conditions

Skin disorders may lower one's quality of life and cause pain. Natural solutions provide a mild and often successful means of treating a range of skin conditions. You will find in this chapter excellent, educational material on using natural therapies for skin disorders, along with instructions on how to utilize them.

**1.Aloe Vera: The Calm Regenerator**
Because of its well-known calming and restorative qualities, aloe vera is a great treatment for cuts, burns, and other skin irritations.

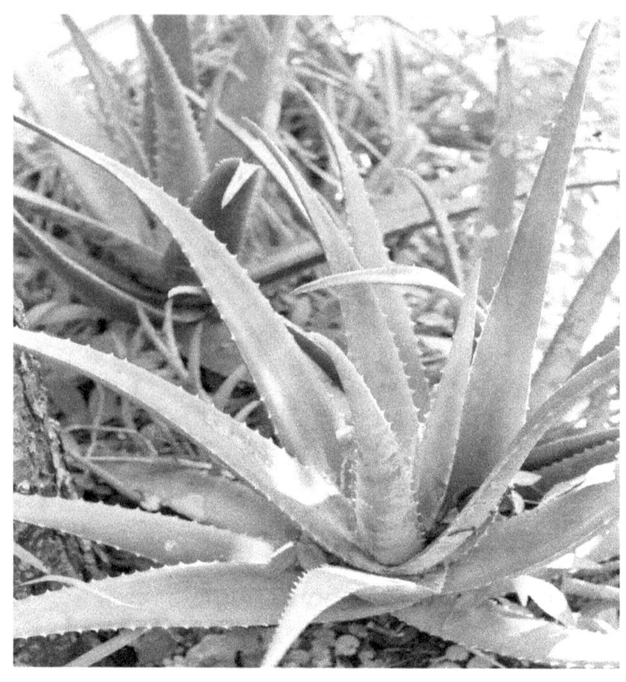

**Method**:
Harvest: Using an aloe vera leaf cutter, cut it off.

**Extract**: Cut open the leaf and remove the transparent gel using a spoon.

**Apply**: Dab the gel onto the region that is afflicted.

**Repeat**: Use two to three times each day till the illness gets better. Tea Tree Oil: The Defender of Antimicrobials

2.Because of its well-known antibacterial and anti-inflammatory qualities, **tea tree oil** is a great choice for the treatment of fungal infections and acne.

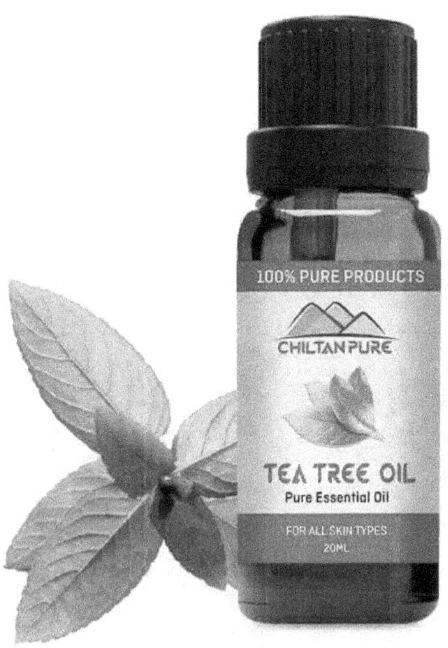


**Method**:
Dilute: Combine a little amount of tea tree oil with coconut oil or other carrier oil.

**To check for an allergic response, apply** a tiny quantity to your forearm and test.

**Apply**: Use a cotton swab to dab the mixture into the afflicted region if there is no response.

**Repetition**: Use once or twice a day until results start to appear.

**3.Muesli**: The Natural Soother Due to its antioxidant and anti-inflammatory qualities, muesli is ideal for relieving dry, irritated, or itchy skin.

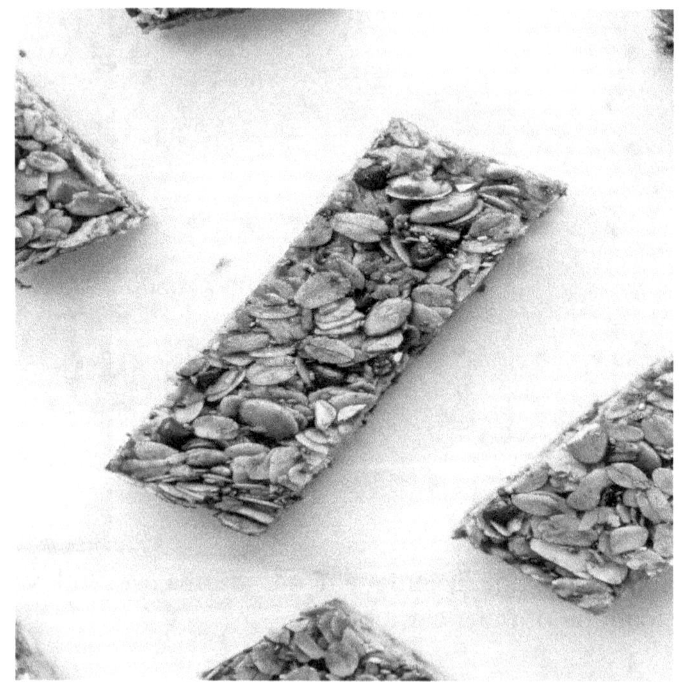

**Method**:
Grind: Using a blender, process plain muesli into a fine powder.

**Mix**: Add the powdered oats to a warm bath.

**Soak**: Give it your all for ten to fifteen minutes.

**wipe Dry**: Use a towel to gently wipe dry your skin.

**4.Honey**: The Sweet Antiseptic Honey is a humectant and natural antiseptic that may aid in the healing of wounds and the moisturization of skin.

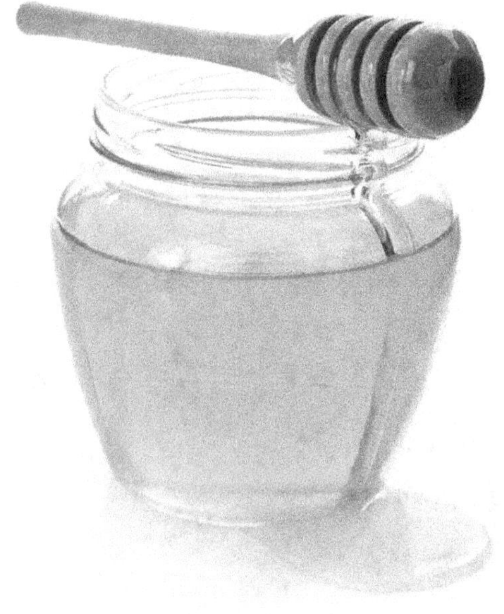

**Method**
**Cleanse**: Use warm water to wash your skin, then pat it dry.

**Apply**: Lightly coat the afflicted region with unprocessed, organic honey.

**Go**: Give the honey fifteen to thirty minutes to settle.

**Rinse**: Use warm water to wash the honey off.

**5.Green Tea**: The Boost to Antioxidants
Rich in antioxidants, green tea helps lessen redness and irritation of the skin.

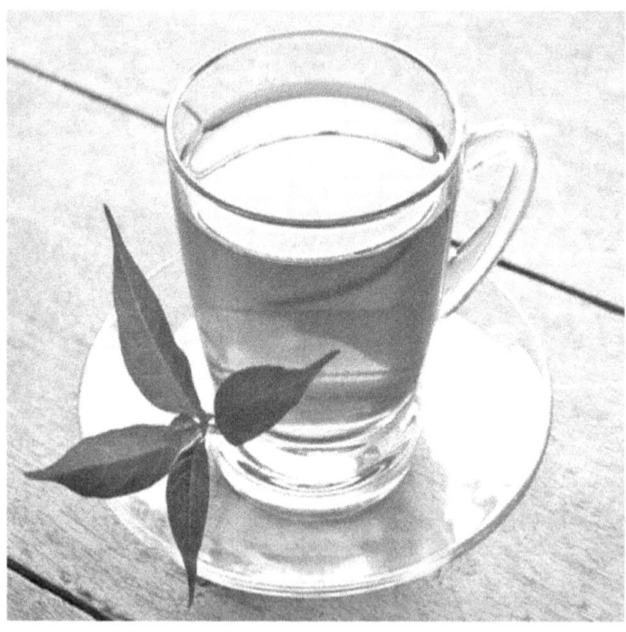

**Method**

**Brew**: Give a green tea bag a three to four-minute steep in boiling water.

**Cool**: Allow the tea bag to reach a temperature that is agreeable.

**Apply**: Press the tea bag gently onto the region that is afflicted.

**Repeat**: For optimal effects, use two to three times a day.

You can simply include these natural treatments into your beauty regimen and they are a tribute to the healing power of nature. Even while they may help with a variety of skin ailments, it's vital to keep in mind that outcomes can differ and that severe or chronic skin problems should be assessed by a medical practitioner.

The goal of this chapter is to provide readers realistic, all-natural skin problem management strategies.

# Herbs for Respiratory Health

Herbs have been utilized for ages to strengthen the lungs and respiratory system since they are vital to general health. This chapter will provide you with excellent and educational information as it examines many herbs that are well-known for their positive benefits on respiratory health.

**1.Schisandra**: The Berry with Five Flavors
Chinese medicine has long used the berry schisandra for its adaptogenic qualities, which support the body's ability to withstand a variety of stresses, particularly those that impact the lungs.

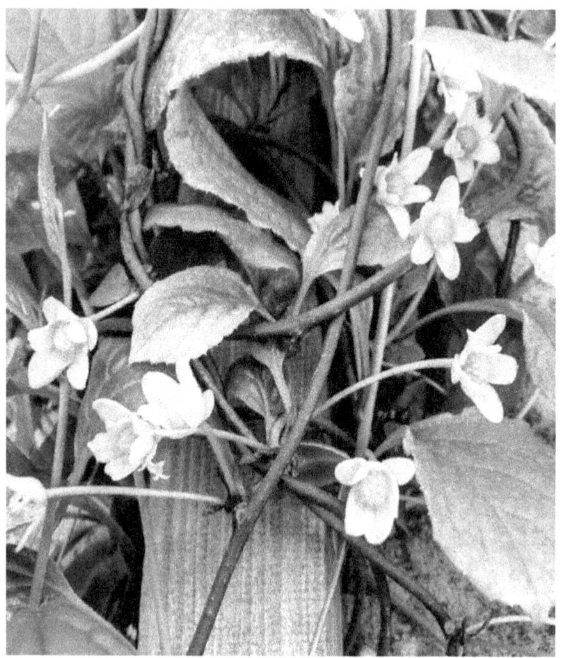

**How to Apply**
**Tea**: In boiling water, brew dried Schisandra berries.

**Supplement**: As prescribed by a healthcare professional, take schizandra capsules.

**2.Yarrow**: The Traditional Inhalation Cure

Yarrow was first used in herbal therapy in ancient Greece, and its history is extensive. It is thought to promote respiratory and lung health.

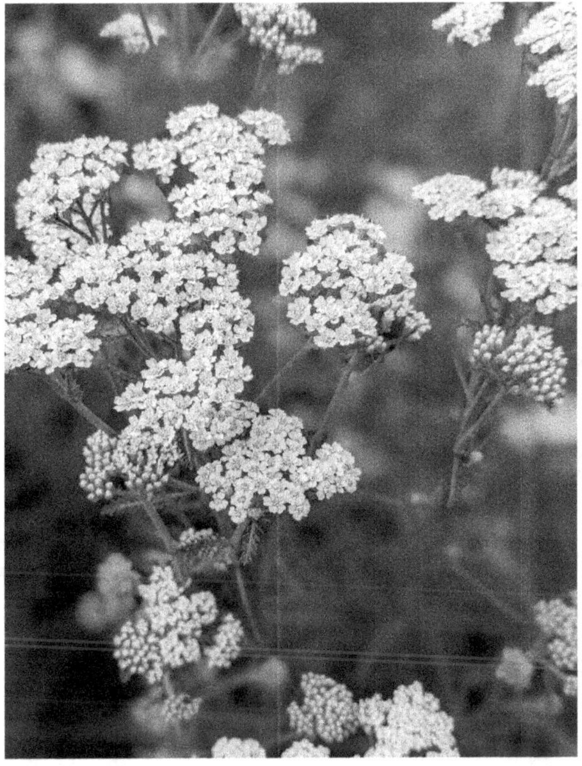

**How to Apply**
Tea: Boil water and steep yarrow blossoms and leaves.

**Tincture**: For respiratory assistance, use a yarrow tincture as prescribed.

**3.Black Seed Oil**: A Strong Seed Reduction
Nigella sativa plant seeds are used to make black seed oil, which is well-known for promoting sinus, respiratory, and lung health.

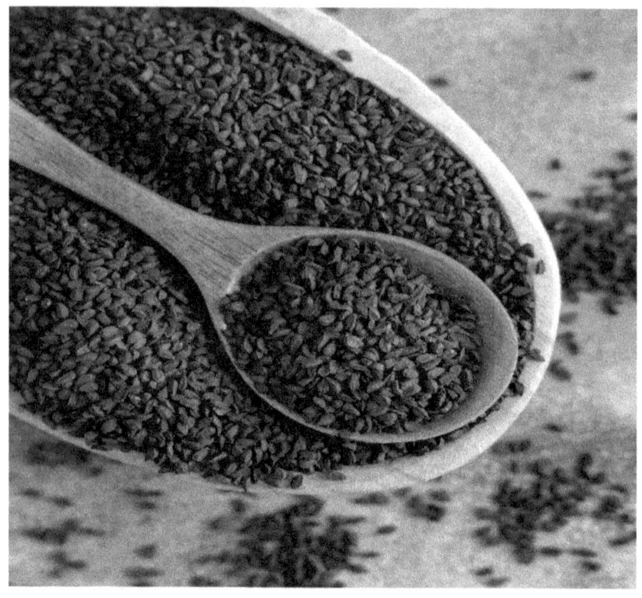

**How to Apply**
Direct: Consume oral cold-pressed black seed oil.

**Mix**: For additional advantages, combine with lemon or honey.

**4.Horehound**: The Anticipating Plant
Horehound is well renowned for helping with phlegm ejection and relieving bronchial problems.

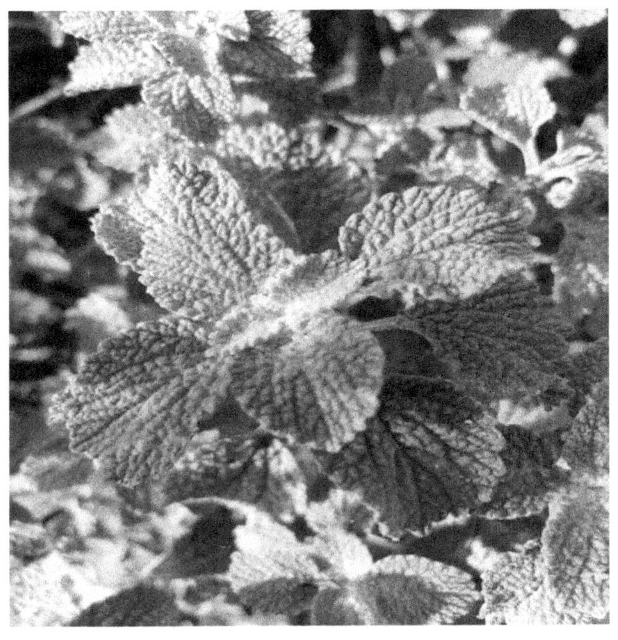

## How to Apply

Syrup: For coughing and congestion, use horehound syrup as prescribed.

**Tea:** To make a calming tea, steep horehound leaves.

**5.Osha Root**: The Herbal Lung

Osha root is highly valued for its capacity to enhance lung oxygenation and is often used to facilitate deep breathing.

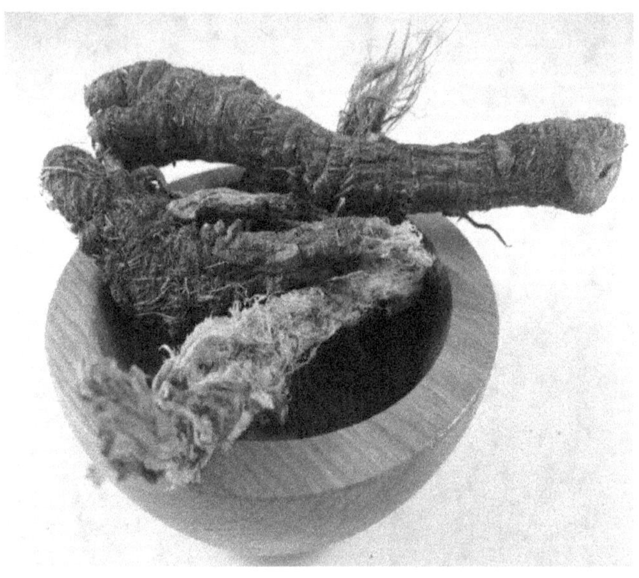

**How to Apply**
Tincture: Administer an osha root tincture as prescribed, particularly in cases of respiratory distress.

**6.Elecampane: The Tonic for Respiration**
Elecampane is well-known for its expectorant qualities, which aid in lung mucus clearance.

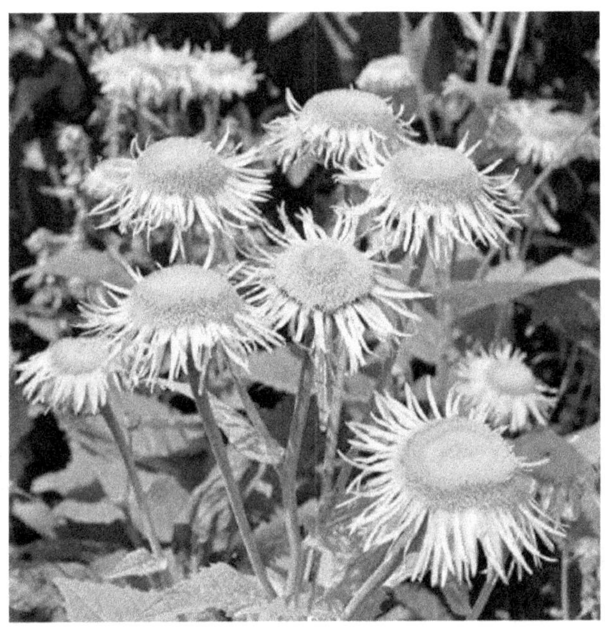

## How to Apply
**Tea**: Brew elecampane root tea by simmering it in water.

**Tincture**: For respiratory assistance, use elecampane tincture.

These herbs provide safe, all-natural means of promoting and preserving respiratory health. To assist strengthen the lungs and improve breathing, they may be administered alone or in combination. Before beginning any new herbal regimen, it is crucial to speak with a healthcare practitioner, particularly if you are taking medication or have pre-existing health concerns.

This chapter offers a thorough analysis of herbs that may promote respiratory health along with helpful suggestions for incorporating them into your daily practice. Anyone interested in learning more about the advantages of herbal medicines will find the information to be both educational and entertaining.

# Managing Pain: Headaches and Joint Pain

An important part of keeping a high quality of life is managing pain. Common illnesses that may vary from little discomfort to incapacitating disorders include headaches and joint pain. You will find excellent, educational material on handling different kinds of pain in this chapter.

### Comprehending Headaches
From tension headaches to migraines, there are many distinct types of headaches and their respective causes. Stress, strained muscles, or more intricate neurological conditions may be the cause1.

### Natural Treatments for Migraines:
**1.Peppermint Oil:** To treat tension headaches, apply a diluted peppermint oil to the temples.

**2.Ginger Tea**: Sip ginger tea to ease headache discomfort and inflammation.

**3.Drink enough water to stay hydrated**; headaches may result from dehydration.

Handling Articular Pain.

**Injuries, overuse, or arthritis may all cause joint discomfort. To properly manage it, it's critical to comprehend the underlying cause.**

**Methods for Relieving Joint Pain**
1.**Cooling Packs**: To relieve discomfort and swelling in the afflicted joint, use ice that has been wrapped in a towel.

**Exercise**: To increase flexibility and strengthen the muscles around your joints, try these low-impact exercises.

**Weight management**: To lessen joint stress, keep your weight within a healthy range.
When to Get Medical Help

**While many joint problems and headaches may be treated at home, other symptoms call for immediate medical attention:**

1.**Headaches**: If you get a sudden, intense headache, blurred vision, or other neurological symptoms, get medical attention.

2.**Joint Pain:** Seek medical attention if the pain is severe, ongoing, or accompanied by warmth and redness surrounding the joint.

A mix of lifestyle modifications, home remedies, and, when required, medical treatments are used in effective pain management.

You may take proactive measures to control your pain and enhance your general well-being by being aware of the causes and remedies for headaches and joint pain.

The purpose of this chapter is to provide readers with useful, all-natural headache and joint pain treatment techniques, expanding their knowledge and giving them the tools they need to take charge of their pain management process.

# CHAPTER 4

# HERBS FOR MENTAL WELL-BEING

## Herbs for Sleep and Insomnia

### Herbs for Mood Improvement

A balanced and meaningful existence depends on mental health. Since ancient times, several herbs have been utilized to promote mental health by providing organic means to elevate mood, lower stress levels, and sharpen cognitive abilities.

### 1.Sage

Sage is well-known for having the ability to improve cognitive function and may help cure Alzheimer's.

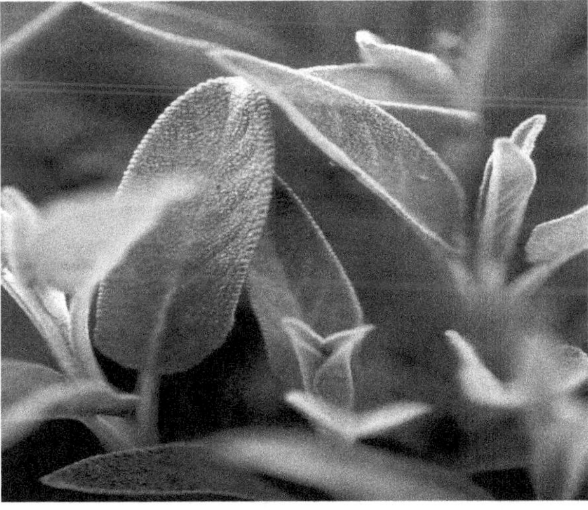

**How to Apply**
**Tea**: Boil one teaspoon of dried sage leaves for five to ten minutes. Enjoy and strain.

**Culinary**: You may include sage in your diet by including it into savory recipes.

**2.Ginseng.**
Ginseng is an adaptogen that may lessen tiredness and enhance mental clarity.

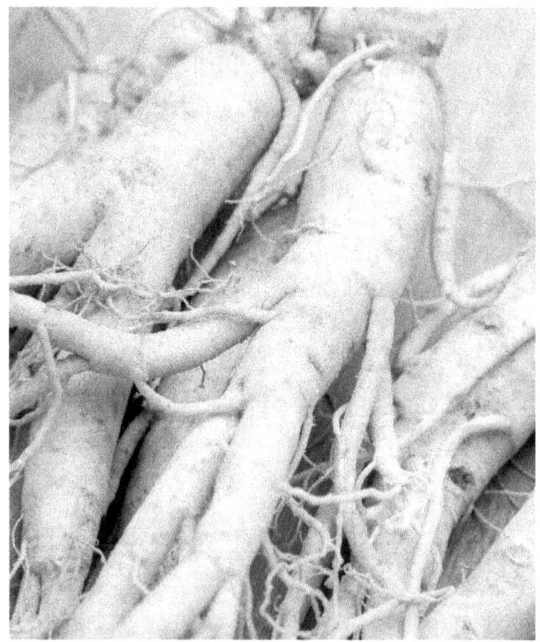

**How to Apply**
**Tea**: Let sliced ginseng root steep in water for ten to fifteen minutes. After chilling, sip.

**Supplement**: Take ginseng pills as prescribed by a physician.
ashwagandha

3.Another adaptogen with a reputation for lowering stress levels is **ashwagandha**.

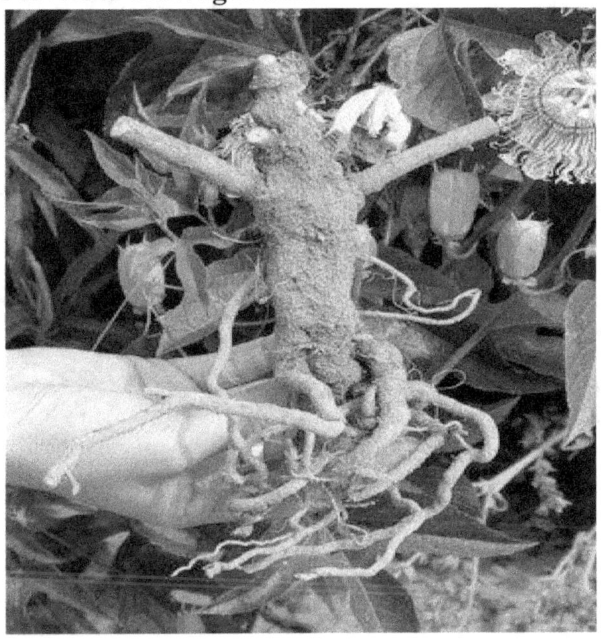

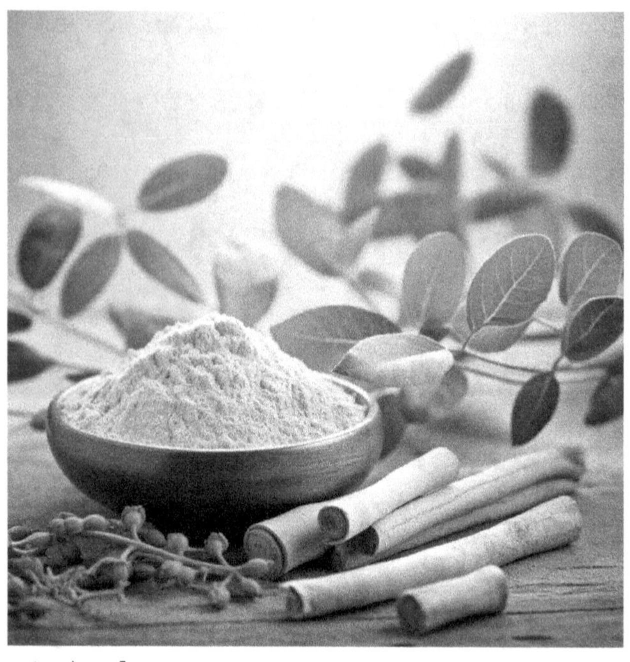

### How to Apply

Powder: Before going to bed, mix ashwagandha powder with warm milk or water.

**Capsule**: Adhere to the dose specified on the supplement label.

### 4.John's Wort

A typical treatment for mild to severe depression is St. John's Wort.

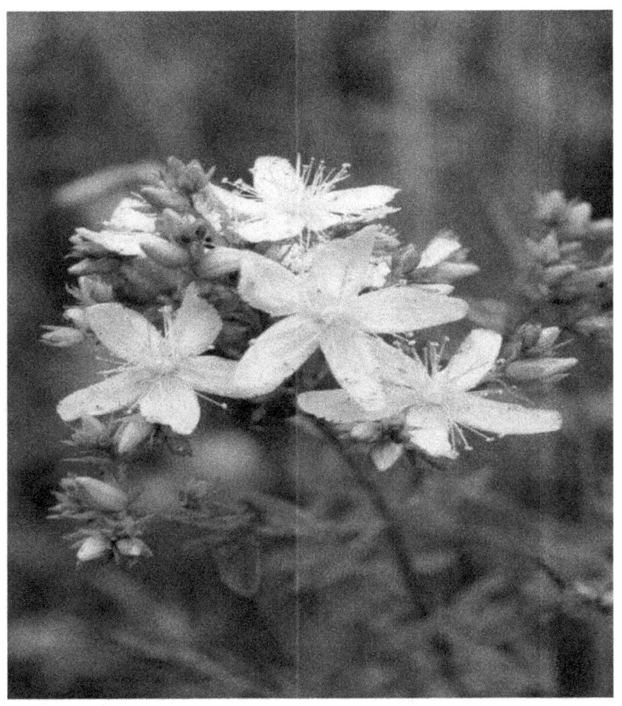

## How to Apply
**Tea**: In boiling water, steep dried St. John's Wort flowers for ten minutes. After straining, sip.

Take supplements as prescribed, but be mindful of any drug interactions.

## Herbs for Restlessness and Sleep
A healthy lifestyle is based on getting enough sleep. The quality of your sleep may be enhanced and relaxation encouraged by the following herbs.

**1.Root of Valerian**
Renowned for its calming properties, Valerian Root is a popular plant for improving sleep.

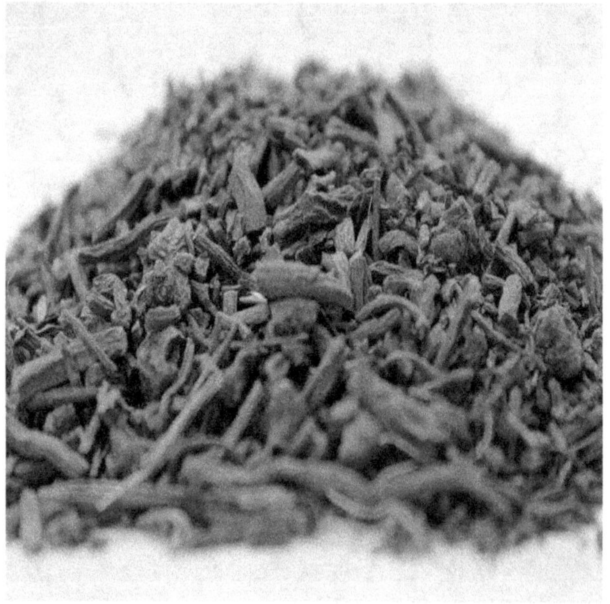

**How to Apply**
**Tea**: In a cup of boiling water, steep one teaspoon of valerian root for ten minutes. Have a drink before going to sleep.

**2.Passionflower**
The relaxing properties of passionflower may enhance sleep.

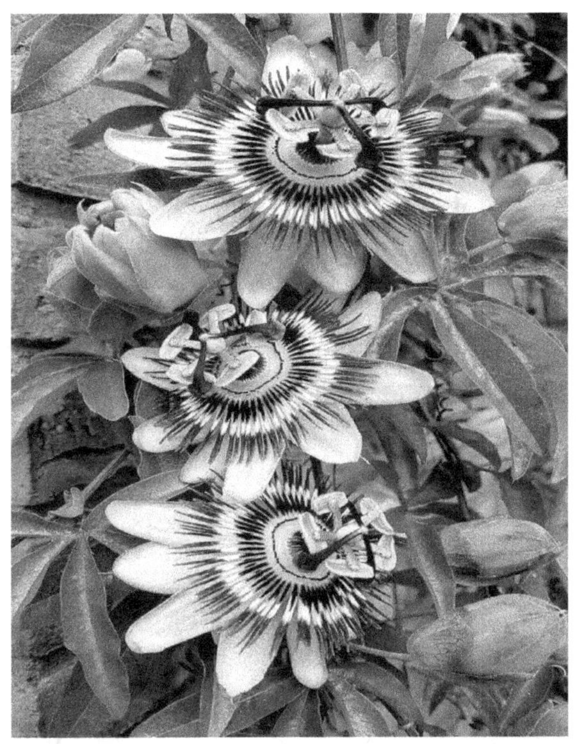

**How to Apply**:
**Tea**: Steep dried passion flower in boiling water for ten minutes.

Have a drink an hour before going to bed.

**Tincture**: Follow the label's instructions for using passionflower tincture.

### 3.Chamomile
A mild plant that might help calm the nervous system and encourage sleep is chamomile.

**How to Apply**
**Tea**: Steep chamomile flowers for five minutes in boiling water. Savor before turning in for the night.

**Inhalation**: Fill your bedroom with a diffuser filled with chamomile essential oil.
Lemon Balm

**4.Lemon balm** may help promote better sleep by lowering tension and anxiety.

**How to Apply**:
**Tea**: Boil some lemon balm leaves for ten minutes. Have a drink at night.

**Topical**: Before going to bed, massage the wrists and temples with lemon balm oil.

Including these herbs in your regular routine may enhance your mental health and help you sleep better. Before beginning any new herbal regimen, always get medical advice, particularly if you are on any drugs or have underlying medical issues.

This chapter offers readers natural ways to improve their quality of life by giving them useful information on herbs that promote sleep and mental health. To guarantee a secure and efficient application, the protocols for using every herb are mentioned.

# Natural Stress Relievers

Although stress is an inherent aspect of life, it may seriously harm our health if it persists for an extended period of time. Thankfully, there are simple, natural methods for reducing stress that may be included into everyday activities. We will look at a number of natural stress relievers in this chapter that support wellbeing and relaxation.

**1.Exercise**
One of the best methods to manage stress is to exercise on a daily basis. Endorphins are natural painkillers and mood enhancers that are released in the brain during exercise.

**How to Include**
**Typical**: On most days of the week, try to get in at least 30 minutes of moderate activity, such as brisk walking or cycling.

**Enjoyment**: To boost the possibility of consistency, choose hobbies you like.

**2.Well-Balanced Diet**
Our emotions are strongly influenced by the foods we consume. The nutrients required to handle stress may be obtained from a diet high in whole foods.

**How to Include**
**Plan**: Make sure your meals include a range of fruits, veggies, lean meats, and healthy grains.

Consume processed meals and foods heavy in sugar and fat in moderation.

### 3.Meditation and Mindfulness

Meditation and mindfulness may ease anxiety, promote relaxation, and enhance focus.

**How to Include**: Regular Routine: Set aside a little period of time each day for meditation or mindfulness.

**Guided Sessions**: If you  are new to meditation, use applications or internet resources for guided meditation.

**4.Sufficient Sleep:** Sufficient sleep is essential for managing stress.
Good sleep may help alleviate stress, whereas inadequate sleep can make it worse.

### How to Include

**Typical**: Create a relaxing atmosphere and stick to a regular sleep routine.

**5.Relaxation**: Before going to bed, read a book or take a warm bath to de-stress.

**6.Social Support** Possessing a robust social network might help protect you from stress.

**7.Speaking** with loved ones might help put things in perspective and provide emotional support.

**How to Include**
**Connect**: Schedule social interaction, even if it's just over the phone or via video chat.

**8.Community**: To meet new people, join organizations or groups that share your interests.

**9.Using aromatherapy**
Using essential oils may help lower stress levels and provide a relaxing effect.

**How to Include**
**Diffuse**: Put sandalwood, chamomile, or lavender oil in an oil diffuser.

**Topical**: To have a relaxing effect, apply diluted essential oils to the pulse points.
Creative Recess

**10.Expressing** emotions and letting go of tension may be therapeutically accomplished via artistic endeavors.

**How to Include: Interests**: Take up artistic endeavors such as writing, painting, or music-making.

**Classes**: Enroll in a workshop or class to pick up new skills and connect with like-minded people.

You may control your stress levels and enhance your general well-being by adopting these all-natural stress relievers into your daily routine. Always keep in mind that you should figure out what works best for you and seek expert assistance if stress gets too much for you.

This chapter offers a comprehensive strategy for handling life's stresses by giving readers doable, all-natural ways to reduce stress. Because of its educational and entertaining design, the material is a great tool for anybody looking to improve their stress-reduction strategies.

# Herbal Aids for Anxiety and Relaxation

Many people look to nature's abundance for solace in their pursuit of peace and mental clarity. Since ancient times, people have used herbal remedies to reduce anxiety and encourage relaxation. We will explore some of the most respected plants in this chapter, which have been supported by both contemporary science and traditional usage.

**1.Lavender**: The Fragrant Soother Known for its calming perfume, lavender is often used in aromatherapy to lower stress and anxiety levels.

**How to Apply**
Aromatherapy: You may inhale straight from the bottle of lavender oil or add a few drops to a diffuser.

**Topical Application:** Blend with a carrier oil and apply to the wrists and temples by massage.

**2.The Calm Root, Valerian Root**
Because of its calming qualities, Valerian root is often used to promote better sleep and lessen anxiety.

**How to Apply**
**Tea**: Ten minutes before going to bed, steep valerian root in hot water.

**Supplement**: As instructed, take one or more capsules of valerian root before going to bed.

**3.The Pacific Elixir, Kava**
Pacific Island civilizations have traditionally used kava for its soothing properties to reduce tension and anxiety.

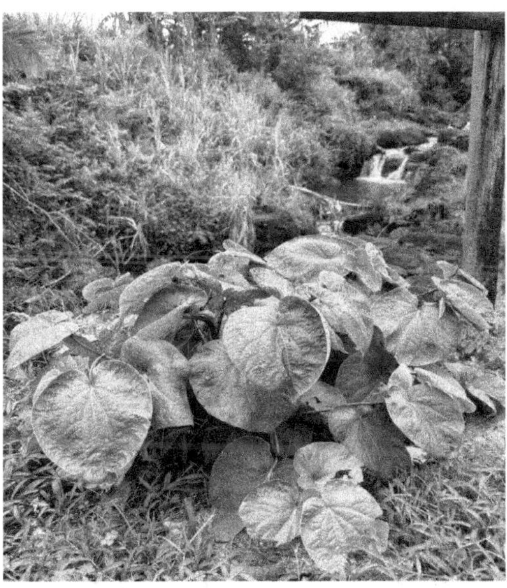

**How to Apply**
**Drink**: Make a kava drink by adding kava powder to water, then straining it out before consuming.

**Supplement**: There are kava supplements available; however, because of the possibility of liver damage, see a physician before taking any.

**4.Passionflower**: The Calming Bloom Due to its gentle sedative properties, passion flower is often used to treat anxiety and insomnia.

**How to Apply**
Tea: Steep dried passion flower in 15 minutes of boiling water.

**Tincture**: As advised, use a few drops of passionflower tincture in water.

**5.Chamomile**: A Calm Nerve Remedy
The mild herb chamomile is well-known for calming anxiety and enhancing the quality of sleep.

**How to Apply**
Tea: In the evening, steep chamomile flowers in hot water for five minutes.

**Supplement**: For anxiety alleviation, use chamomile capsules as prescribed.

**6.Ashwagandha**: The Herbal Combatant

An adaptogen called ashwagandha may alleviate anxiety symptoms and assist the body in regulating stress.

**How to Apply**
**Powder**: Add ashwagandha powder to warm water or milk, then stir and enjoy.

**Ashwagandha capsules:** Take them in accordance with the suggested dose.

**7.St. John's Wort The Mood Uplifter**
Commonly used to treat mild to severe depression, St. John's Wort may also be helpful for anxiety.

**How to Apply:**
Tea: Brew the dry herb in a cup of hot water once or twice a day.

**Supplement**: Liquid extracts and pills containing St. John's Wort are available.

These herbal remedies provide a healthy way to promote calmness and manage anxiety. Herbal treatments may be beneficial, but it's important to speak with a doctor before beginning any, particularly if you  are also on other drugs. Herbs can interfere with other medications. These herbs might be a useful supplement to your health regimen if used under the right supervision.

This chapter gives readers a comprehensive review of herbal remedies for anxiety and relaxation, giving them insight into non-invasive ways to improve their mental health. Because of the material's approachable and captivating form, it might be a helpful tool for those looking for other ways to manage their stress.

# CHAPTER 5

# SPECIALIZED HERBAL APPLICATIONS

## Women's Health: Herbs for Hormonal Balance

**Specific Uses of Herbs**

An essential component of women's health, hormonal balance affects everything from mood and general wellbeing to the menstrual cycle. Herbal remedies have long been utilized to maintain hormonal balance. We will look at a few of these plants and their uses in this chapter.

**1.Nigella sativa, or Nigella seeds**

Nicknamed nigella seeds, or fennel flower, or kalonji, are high in antioxidants and contain thymoquinone, which may have the ability to balance hormones.

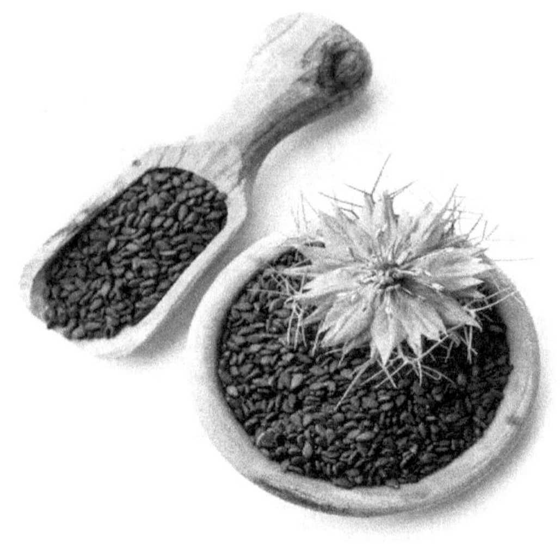

## 2. Vitex (Agnus-castus Vitex)

Vitex, sometimes referred to as chaste berry, is a well-known plant that acts on the pituitary gland to help control the menstrual cycle, alleviate PMS symptoms, and enhance fertility.

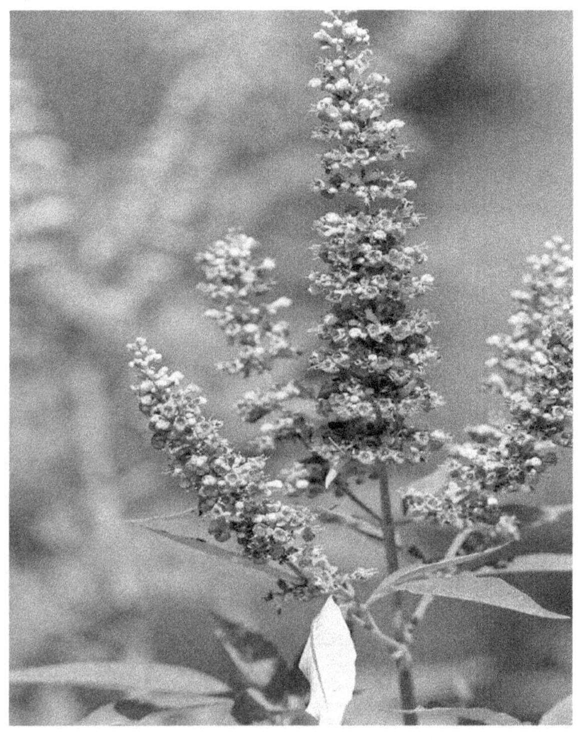

### 3.Nettle Leaf (Urtica dioica) with Stinging

The capacity of nettle leaf to promote liver health is well known; hormone balance depends on liver function. Moreover, it could decrease DHT, a hormone connected to hair loss.

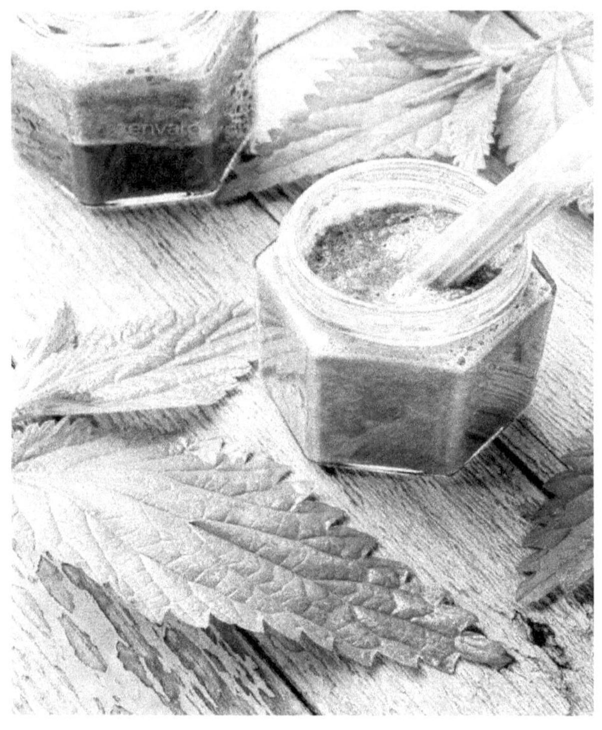

## 4.(Matricaria ) chamomile

Not only does chamomile aid with relaxation and sleep, but it may also lower testosterone levels and help control blood sugar, which can be helpful for disorders like PCOS.

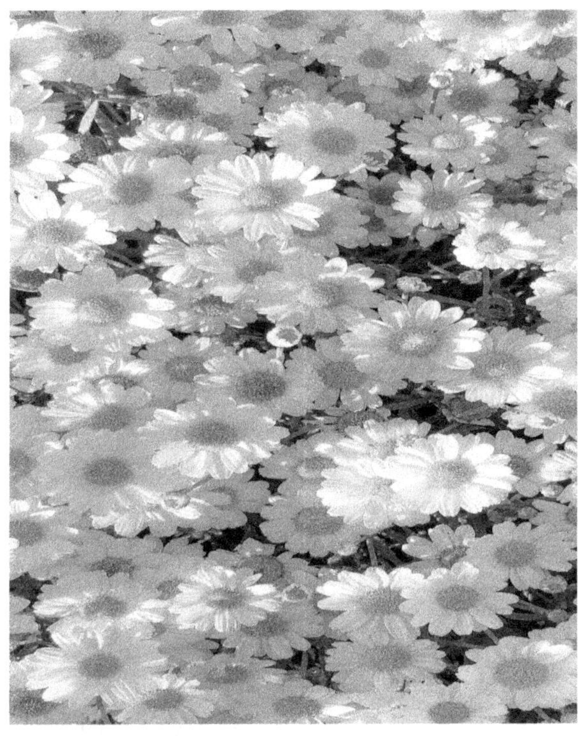

**5.The Trifolium pratense**, or red clover
Isoflavones, which are plant-based substances that resemble estrogen and may aid with PMS and menopausal symptoms, are found in red clover.

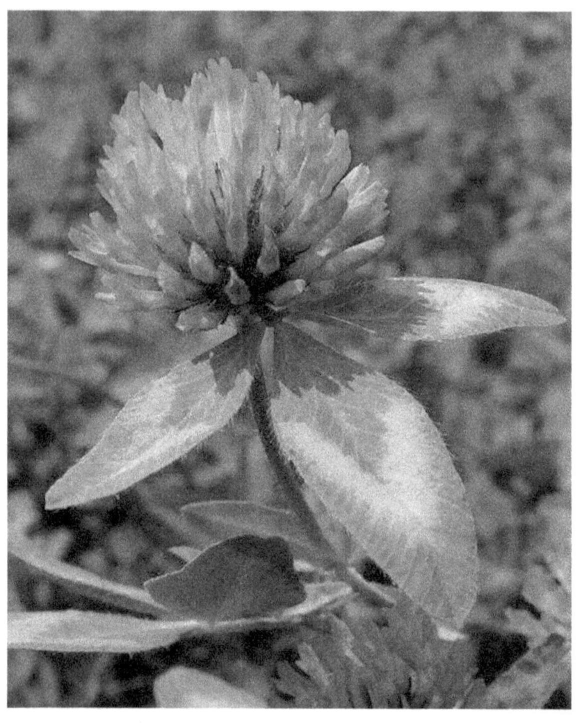

### 6.The Berry Schisandra (Schisandra )

Because of its adaptogenic qualities, schisandra berries may help maintain hormonal balance and stress resilience.

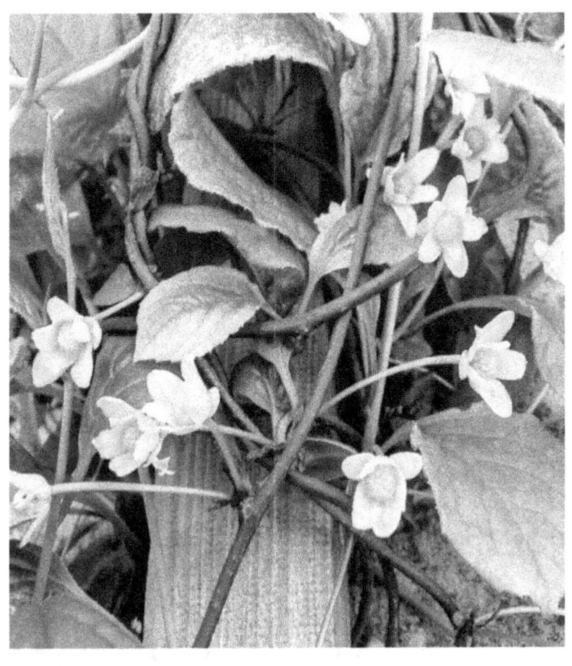

## 7.Paeonia , or peonies

In traditional medicine, peonies have been used to improve hormonal balance and may be helpful with disorders like PCOS.

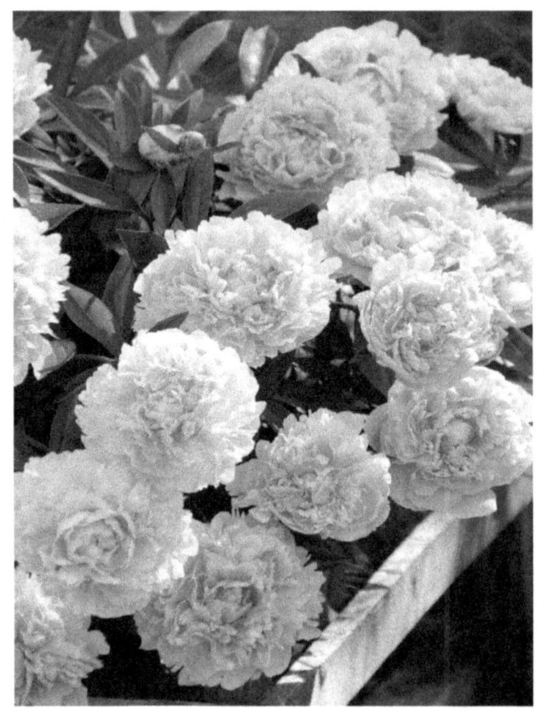

**8.Actaea , or black cohosh,**
Black cohosh is often used to treat mood swings and hot flashes associated with menopause.

**Including Herbs in Your Daily Teas**: Use tea bags or dried herbs to brew herbal teas.

**Supplements**: Take tinctures or capsules as prescribed by a physician.

**Topical**: Apply these herbs on your skin as oils or creams.

**Safety and Things to Think About**

Herbs are a valuable ally in regulating hormonal health, but they must be taken sparingly. Before beginning any new herbal regimen, always get advice from a healthcare professional, particularly if you are expecting, nursing, or have a medical problem. Be mindful of possible conflicts between prescription drugs and other dietary supplements.

An overview of herbs that may help women's health by balancing their hormones is given in this chapter. The information is intended to be both educational and useful, providing herbal cures as natural options for anyone looking to improve their health.

# Men's Health: Herbs for Vitality and Well-being

Men who want to be healthy and vibrant typically look for natural remedies that fit within a holistic perspective. For decades, men's health has been supported by herbs in a number of ways, such as energy levels, hormone balance, and general vitality.

This chapter will highlight herbs that are especially good for men's health and provide use guidelines.

**1.Serenoa , or palmetto.**

Renowned for promoting prostate health, saw palmetto may help treat benign prostatic hyperplasia (BPH).

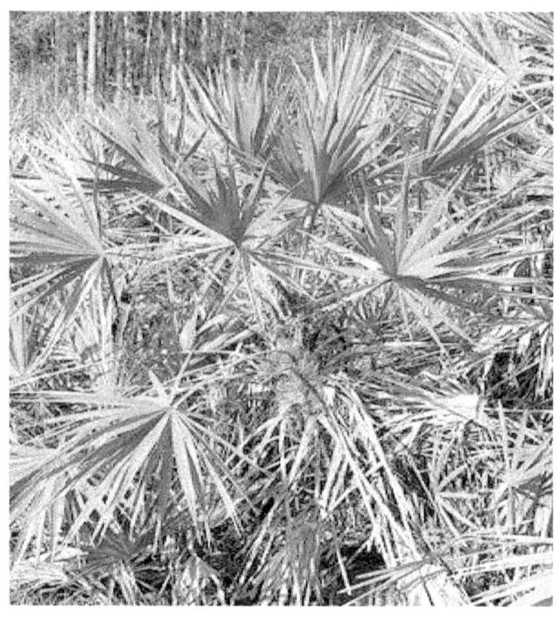

**Method: Capsules**: Saw palmetto is usually taken as capsules, with the manufacturer recommending a dosage.

**Tea**: Another option, however less popular, is to steep the dried berries to produce a tea.

### 2.Ashwagandha (Indica brevis)
Ashwagandha is an adaptogen that may increase energy and mental clarity while assisting the body in reducing stress.

**Method**:
**Powder**: Take one teaspoon of ashwagandha powder once a day in a glass of warm milk or water.

**For capsules**, adhere to the dose recommendations on the supplement's packaging.

3.**Ginseng, or ginger** is another adaptogen that has been shown to increase energy and decrease fatigue.

**Method**: To make tea, simmer thinly sliced ginseng root in water for fifteen minutes or so, then sip the resulting infusion.

**Supplement**: Follow the directions on the product package when taking ginseng pills or capsules.

4.**Maca Root (Lepidium )** is often used to enhance sexual function, increase libido, and raise energy levels.

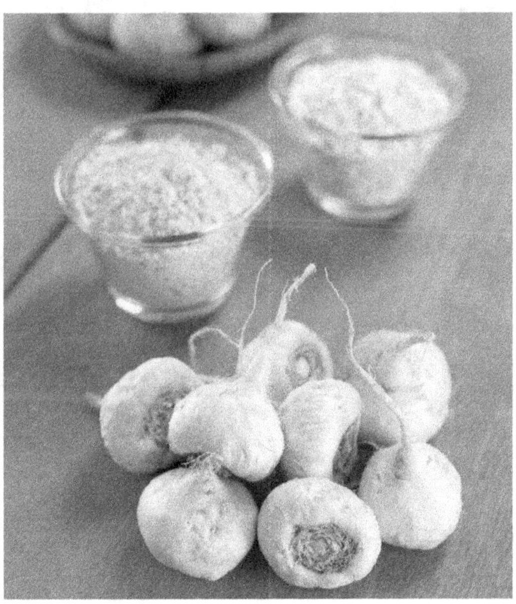

**Method**
**Powder**: You may add maca root powder to yogurt, muesli and smoothies.

**Maca root capsules**: Take them as directed by the manufacturer.

**5.Urtica** , or nettle root, has been shown to improve prostate health and lessen BPH symptoms.

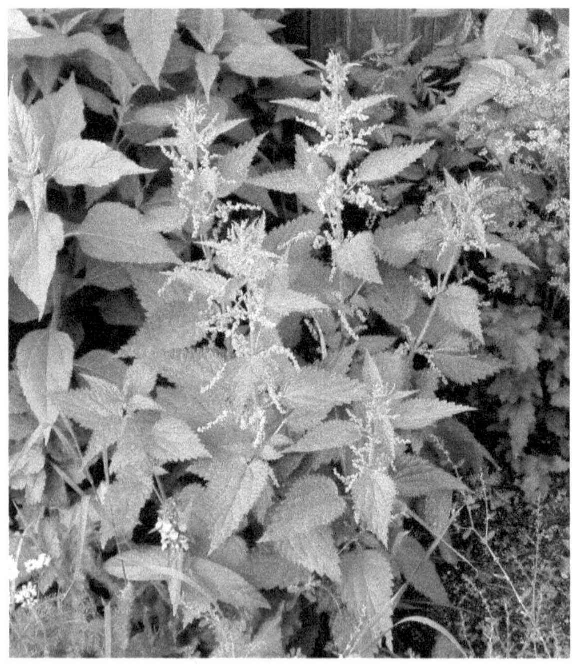

**Method**: To make nettle root tea, steep it in boiling water for ten to fifteen minutes.

**Tincture**: Follow the directions on the nettle root tincture and add it to water.

**6.Trigonella** foenum-graecum, or fenugreek
Studies have looked at fenugreek's ability to raise testosterone levels and promote better metabolic health.

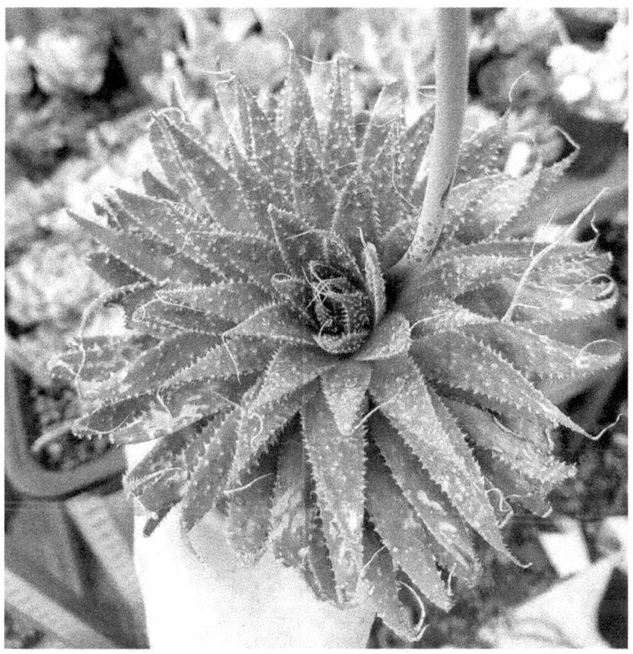

**Method: Seeds**: Either include soaked fenugreek seeds into meals or chew on them.

**Supplement**: Follow the directions on the fenugreek supplement packet.

**7.Curry powder (Curcuma longa)**
Curcumin, an anti-inflammatory compound found in turmeric, may improve joint health and lessen inflammation.

**Method: Cooking**: Add turmeric powder to your food for flavor and health advantages.

**Supplement**: Take supplements containing curcumin as recommended; to improve absorption, black pepper extract is often added.

**8.Rose Rhodiola**
It is thought that rhodiola rosea enhances both physical and mental vigor, particularly under stressful and exhausting situations.

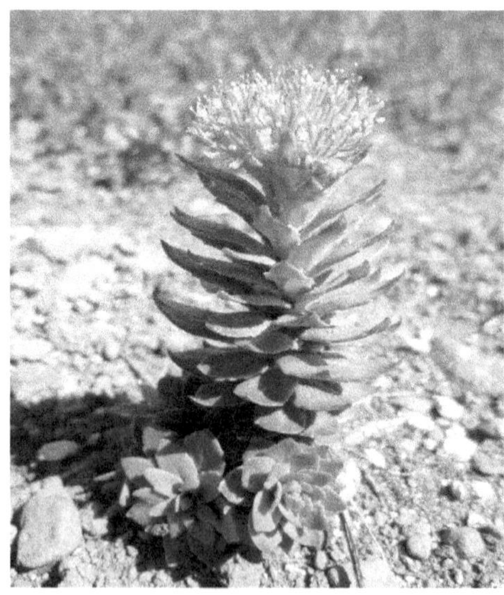

**Method**
**Tea**: To make tea, steep rhodiola rosea in hot water.

Rhodiola rosea capsules should be taken as directed on the product label.

These herbs provide a non-invasive way to improve the health and energy of men. Herbs may interfere with pharmaceuticals, so it's crucial to speak with a healthcare professional before beginning any new herbal regimen, particularly for those with pre-existing medical disorders or those on medication. These herbs may be a useful complement to a holistic health plan when used under the right supervision.

# Herbal Care for Children and the Elderly

Both children's and the elderly's health and well-being may be greatly enhanced by herbal treatment. But, it's crucial to use awareness and care while using herbal treatments, particularly for these vulnerable populations. High-quality, educational information about safe and efficient herbal care for kids and seniors, along with use instructions, will be included in this chapter.

### Children's Herbal Care
Because of their heightened sensitivity, children react strongly to mild herbs while stronger herbs may have unintended effects. It is crucial to use plants with a long history of traditional usage and gentleness.

**Herbs that Are Safe for Kids**
1.**Chamomile (Matricaria** ): Reduces anxiety and promotes restful sleep.

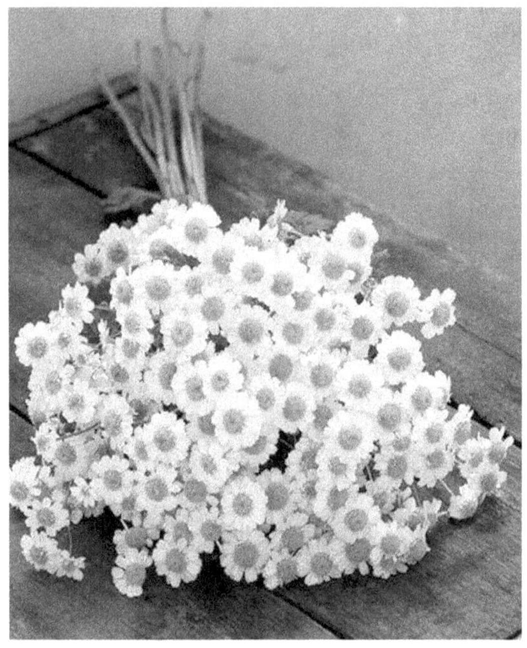

**2.Lemon balm**
Melissa officinalis, also known as lemon balm, soothes the nervous system and reduces restlessness.

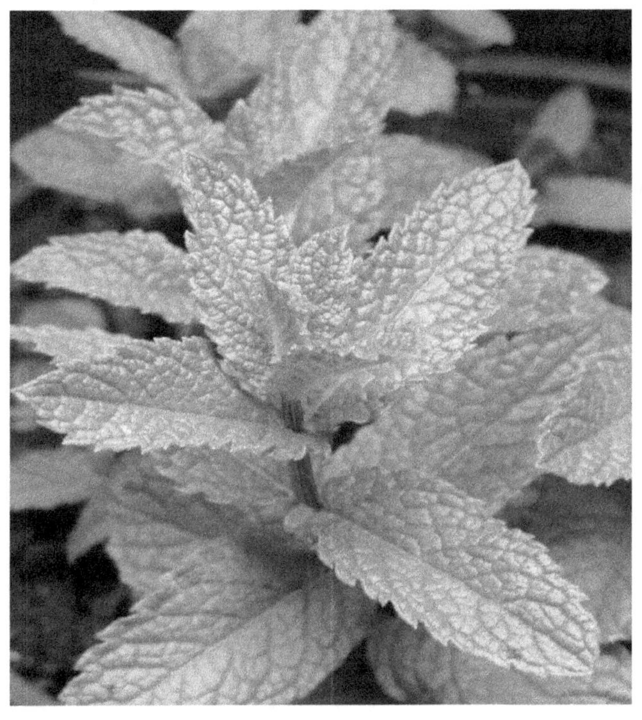

### 3.Echinacea

**Echinacea**: The immune system is supported by Echinacea spp.

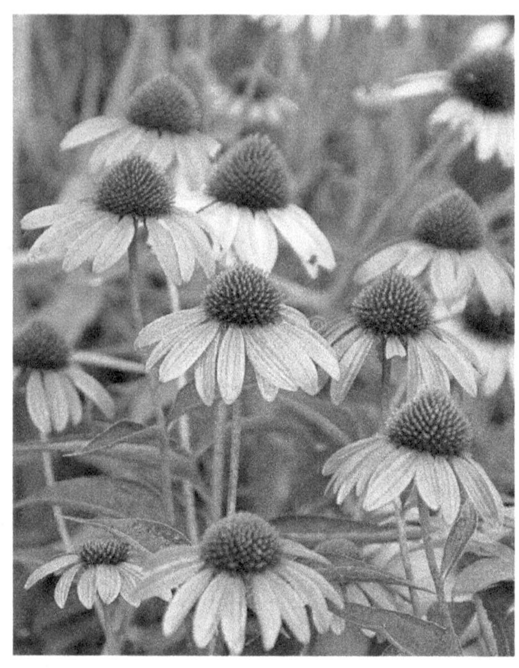

**Method**:

**Teas**: Use these herbs to make a mild tea that kids may sip.

**Topical**: Apply diluted herbal lotions or oils to your skin.

**Form of dosage**

**Dosage**: Always utilize a pediatric herbalist or healthcare professional for advice, and always take lesser amounts than those for adults.

**Herbal Remedies for Seniors**

It's important to take into account possible herb-drug interactions since senior people may take many drugs and have different health issues. Herbs are to supplement mainstream medicine, not take its place.

**1.Zingiber , or ginger**, eases inflammation and promotes better digestion.

**2.Ginkgo (Ginkgo biloba)**: Promotes circulation and mental clarity.

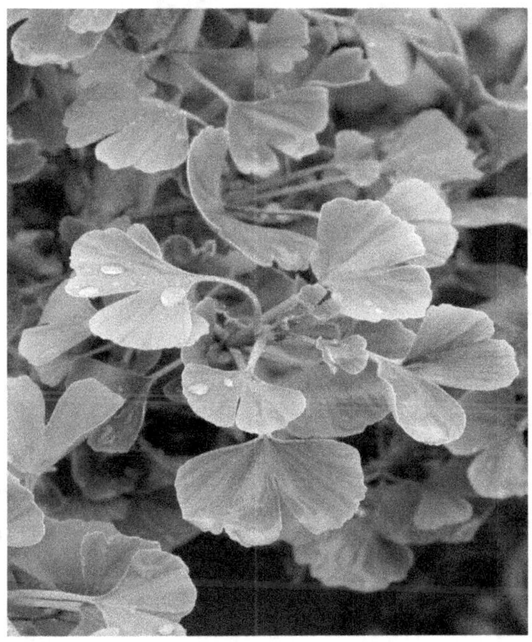

**3.Ginger**
Curcuma longa, or turmeric, has anti-inflammatory qualities that are good for joints.

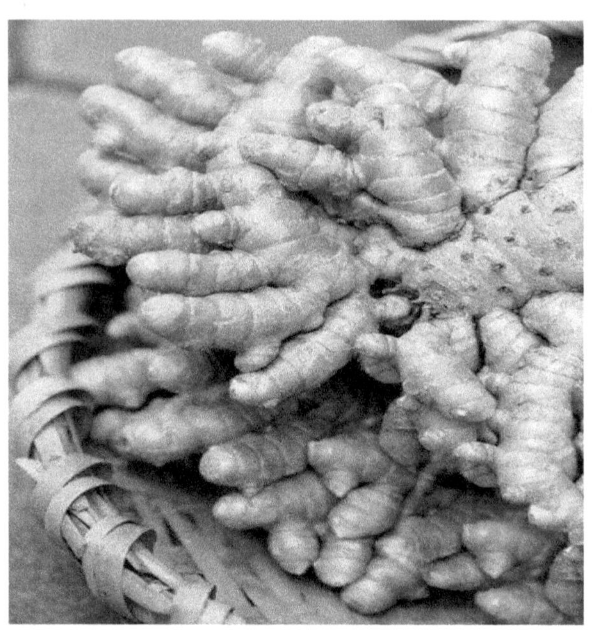

## Method

Blending in

**Infusions**: Make infusions with these herbs so that senior citizens may drink them all day long.

**Supplements**: If tea or infusion is not to your taste, think about taking herbal supplements, but only under a doctor's supervision.

**Consultation**: Before beginning any new herbal regimen, particularly for those using other drugs, always get advice from a healthcare professional.

**Basic Standards for the Quality of Herbal Care**: Use premium, organic herbs to guarantee their strength and purity.

**Consultation:** Before using herbs, especially for young patients or the elderly, get counsel from a licensed herbalist or healthcare professional.

**Instruction**
**Education**: Inform carers and yourself on the appropriate use of herbs, including doses and any adverse effects.

A basic grasp of herbal treatment for children and the elderly is given in this chapter, with a focus on safety, appropriate doses, and the value of expert advice. The information is designed to be both useful and educational, providing natural solutions for anybody looking to improve the health of these at-risk groups.

# CHAPTER 6

# CREATING HERBAL FORMULAS

## Blending Herbs for Specific Conditions

Combining Herbs for Particular Illnesses
Herbal formula creation is a science and an art that requires a thorough knowledge of each particular plant and the illnesses it may treat. You will learn how to make herbal mixes that are useful for certain health concerns in this chapter.

**Comprehending Herbal Properties**
It's important to know the characteristics of the herbs and how they work together before mixing them. Herbs may be adaptogenic, analgesic, or anti-inflammatory, among other effects. By being aware of these characteristics, you may choose herbs that work well together and increase the formula's overall potency.

**The Method of Blending**
**Determine the Main Action**: Identify the formula's primary emphasis. Is it to aid in digestion, reduce pain, or maybe strengthen the immune system? Based on this main action, choose your lead herb. Select Supporting Herbs: Include herbs that amplify and reinforce the activity of the main herb.

These need to have ancillary advantages that complement the objectives of the formula.

**Take Synergists and Drivers into Account**: Add herbs that aid in improving the formula's absorption and directing its effects to the intended bodily region.

**Equilibrate the Formula:** To make the mix more appetizing and harmonic, make sure it is balanced not just in terms of herbal effects but also in flavor and energy.

**Creating Formulas for Particular Situations**
**Problems with the Digestive System**: To help ease the digestive system, combine carminatives like peppermint with bitter plants like dandelions .

**Stress and Anxiety**: To help with relaxation and stress resistance, combine nervines like lemon balm with adaptogens like ashwagandha.

**Immune Support**: To strengthen the body's natural defenses, combine lymphatic herbs like calendula with immune stimulants like echinacea.

**Dosage and Management**
**Teas**: Steep the herbs in boiling water to make herbal teas for a mild impact.

**Tinctures**: Use glycerin- or alcohol-based tinctures for a more concentrated dosage.

Encapsulate the powdered herbs for ease of use and regulated dosing.

**Safety and Precautions**
**Talking with:** When making formulae for young patients, the elderly, or those with complicated medical issues, it is always advisable to get the advice of a trained herbalist or healthcare professional.

**Allergies and Interactions**: Recognise any possible allergies and how they could affect other supplements or prescription drugs.

**Quality**: To guarantee the purity and efficacy of your solution, choose premium, organic herbs.

A basic concept of creating herbal formulae for certain health issues is given in this chapter. The text highlights the significance of knowledge, equilibrium, and safety throughout the blending process, providing readers with the necessary resources to create custom herbal treatments.

# Dosage Guidelines for Safe Use

Following the recommended dose amounts is essential when taking herbal treatments to guarantee both safety and efficacy. The body may be strongly affected by the active chemicals in herbs, making them powerful substances.

The following are some general rules to abide by:

**1. Start with Small Doses:** Take the lowest amount that is advised at first and see how your body reacts. If required, you may progressively raise the dose; nonetheless, you should never go above the suggested limit.

**2. Adhere to the Directions**: Make sure you utilize herbs in accordance with the directions provided by a healthcare provider or on the product label. This covers the dosage, how often it is taken, and how long it is used for.

**3. Take into Account the Form**: The dose may change depending on the herb's form (tea, tincture, tablet, etc.). For example, you will need less tincture since it's more concentrated than tea.

**4. Age Matters:** Depending on age, dosages may change. Because of their smaller bodies and slower metabolic rates, children and the elderly usually need lower doses.

**5. Recognise Interactions**: Certain plants may interfere with prescription drugs or other herbal remedies. Speak with a healthcare professional to prevent negative interactions.

**6. Listen to Your Body**: Be Aware of Any Adverse Reactions or Side Effects. Stop taking the herb and see a doctor if you feel any pain.

**7. Quality Matters:** Make use of respectable, high-quality brands. In addition to being useless, low-quality plants may include toxic metals or pesticides.

**8. Storage and Shelf Life:** Keep herbs dry and cold, and pay attention to when they expire. Certain herbs may deteriorate and lose their potency over time.

**9. Pregnancy and Nursing**: Pregnancy and nursing are two times when a lot of herbs should be avoided. A healthcare professional should always be consulted before using.

**10. Chronic Conditions**: Before utilizing herbal medicines, speak with your doctor if you have a chronic illness or are on prescription medication.

Recall that safety does not necessarily equate to natural. It's essential to take herbal treatments sensibly and to be aware of any possible side effects.

## Customizing Remedies for Individual Needs

Since each person is different, so too is the way our bodies react to herbal therapies. An essential component of successful herbal therapy is tailoring remedies to each patient's unique health demands. When customizing herbal treatments to meet the needs of each person, keep the following factors in mind:

**1. Personal Health History**: It's critical to have a complete awareness of one's medical history, including previous illnesses, surgeries, and long-term diseases. This information may be used to determine whether plants are potentially dangerous or useful.

**2. Biochemical Individuality**: Everybody is different in terms of their biochemistry. The way that one reacts to certain herbs may be influenced by a number of factors, including diet, metabolism, and heredity.

**3. Current Medication:** Because herbs might interact with medications and supplements, it's important to take them into account.

**4. Lifestyle Factors:** A person's diet, exercise routine, stress level, and sleep habits may all have an impact on their health and the selection and efficacy of herbal medicines.

**5. Allergies and Sensitivities: To** prevent negative responses, be mindful of any known allergies or sensitivities.

**6. Age and Life Stage:** The choice and dose of herbs might be influenced by age-related changes as well as life phases like puberty, pregnancy, or menopause.

**7. Cultural Practices**: Including cultural customs and beliefs may improve herbal treatments' acceptability and efficacy.

**8. flavor and Preference:** For long-term compliance and pleasure, the remedy's flavor and form (tea, tincture, or pill) should be taken into account.

**9. Observation and Feedback**: It's important to regularly observe and provide feedback. The person's reaction should be taken into account while modifying the therapies.

**10. Professional Advice**: Speaking with a licensed herbalist or medical professional may provide guidance on developing a customized herbal regimen.

Herbal medicines may be customized to an individual's unique health requirements, preferences, and circumstances by taking these aspects into account. This results in improved health outcomes and a more individualized approach to wellbeing.

# CHAPTER 7

# ADVANCED HERBAL TECHNIQUES

## Sophisticated Methods of Extraction

If you want to learn more about the art of herbalism, knowing how to extract herbs with precision will greatly increase the strength and effectiveness of your own cures. As they have more skill, novices may want to try these advanced methods:

**1.Supercritical Fluid Extraction (SFE):**This technique extracts active components from plants by using supercritical carbon dioxide. SFE is renowned for its effectiveness and capacity to protect sensitive chemicals from heat-related degradation.

**2.Ultrasonic-Assisted Extraction (UAE)**
This method releases active chemicals into the extraction solvent by agitating the plant material using ultrasonic vibrations. It's a rapid process that may produce extracts with a lot of power.

**3. Microwave-Assisted Extraction (MAE)** This technique speeds up the extraction process by heating the plant material and solvent using microwave radiation. In particular, this technique may be helpful for extracting substances that are soluble in water.

**4. Soxhlet Extraction:** A more conventional method, Soxhlet extraction extracts chemicals from plant materials by repeatedly washing them in a solvent. It is particularly helpful for substances that are not very soluble in the solvent.

**5. Enfleurage:** This technique, which is often used in fragrance, is applying fresh petals to a glass surface that has been lightly oiled with fat. The essential oils from the petals are gradually absorbed by the fat.

**6. Spagyric Extraction**: In this alchemical procedure, the plant material is fermented before the mineral components are extracted and distilled from the burned plant ash. The goal of this all-encompassing method is to fully extract the plant's essence.

These sophisticated methods need careful consideration of knowledge, tools, and safety. Novices should proceed cautiously while using these techniques and, if at all feasible, consult experienced herbalists for advice.

# Long-term Preservation of Herbal Remedies

Maintaining the purity and strength of herbal treatments over time is crucial to guaranteeing their efficacy when required.

**1. Drying**: One of the oldest and most reliable ways to preserve herbs is by drying them. Herbs that are dried properly may keep their efficacy for many years. It's important to dry them rapidly to stop mold from growing, yet gently to keep their volatile oils intact.

**2. Tincturing**: Herbs are soaked in alcohol to create tinctures, which are concentrated herbal extracts. This process not only extracts strong, non-water soluble chemicals from the plants but also preserves them for many years.

**3. Freezing**: Certain herbs, particularly those that don't dry well, may retain their freshness by freezing. It's crucial to remember, however, that freezing may change certain plants' texture.

**4. Canning**: Herbal vinegars and syrups may be canned to preserve them. This entails sterilizing jars and heating the preparations to a certain temperature.

**5. Oil Infusions**: To make salves and ointments, herbs may be infused into oils. The oil prolongs the herbal properties' shelf life by acting as a preservative.

**6. Honey Infusions**: Honey may be used to create oxymels, a concoction of honey and vinegar, and herbal honeys. Honey is a natural preservative. If stored correctly, these preparations may be kept for many years.

**7. Glycerites**: Glycerites are a sugary substitute for those who abstain from alcohol. They may last up to two years and are created by extracting herbal ingredients with glycerin.

**8. Appropriate Storage:** Whichever approach you use, careful storage is essential. Herbs need to be stored somewhere dry, dark, and cold. Airtight lidded glass containers are the best option for keeping out light and moisture.

**9. Labeling:** Make sure to include the anticipated shelf life and the preparation date on all of your medicines' labels. This makes it easier to monitor their safety and potency over time.

**10. Regular Inspection**: Keep an eye out for any indications of spoiling, like mold, strange smells, or discoloration, on any medicines that have been stored.

You may keep a home apothecary that endures and is prepared to promote health and wellbeing when needed by adhering to these preservation procedures.

This area is designed to provide novices interested in herbal home cures high-quality, educational material.
It is important to encourage readers, particularly those with medical issues or on medication, to always get advice from a healthcare expert prior to consuming or producing herbal treatments.

# Wildcrafting: Ethical Foraging and Identification

Gathering plants for food or medicine from their natural environment is a joyful hobby known as "wildcrafting," which helps us feel more connected to the natural world and our ancestors. But it's important to approach wildcrafting with awareness and respect.

**1. Know the Laws**: Become acquainted with local laws before going foraging. Laws safeguarding certain plant species or habitats exist in several places.

**2. certain Identification:** Prior to harvesting, you should always be absolutely certain of a plant's identification. Utilize seminars, applications, or field guides to learn about the traits of plants.

**3. Sustainable Harvesting**: Only remove what is necessary, leaving enough for the plant to flourish. Never capture rare or endangered species, and refrain from overharvesting.

**4. Timing Is Everything**: For maximum efficacy, harvest plants at the appropriate time of year. For instance, when the plant stores its energy underground in the autumn, it is usually ideal to harvest its roots.

**5. Get Permission** First: Ask the landowner for permission before foraging on their property. Honor the earth and the kindness of those who let you forage.

**6. Leave No Trace**: Reduce the amount of damage you do to the environment. Keep to the walkways, don't step on any plants, and pick up after yourself.

**7. Ethical Considerations:** Take into account the cultural importance of plants to local or indigenous populations. Certain plants could be considered holy or essential to their customs.

**8. Personal Safety**: Pay attention to your surroundings and any possible dangers, including animals, dangerous plants, and borders of private property.

**9. Share Knowledge**: Teach people about ethics and foraging techniques. It will be better protected for future generations the more people appreciate and understand nature.

**10. Never Stop Learning**: Keep up with ecological shifts and conservation initiatives that might have an impact on plant populations.

Wildcrafting may be a sustainable activity that improves our lives and strengthens our connection with the environment if we go by these rules.

For novices, this part is designed to be both educational and entertaining, giving them the basic information they need to begin ethical wildcrafting. It's crucial to remind readers that, even though it may be a fun activity, foraging requires consideration for the environment as well as local laws and traditions.

# CHAPTER 8

# BUILDING A HOLISTIC LIFESTYLE

## Integrating Herbal Remedies into Daily Life

For individuals starting on a herbal home remedy path, living a holistic lifestyle means incorporating health into all facets of your life rather than simply treating illnesses.

**1.Begin with Minor Adjustments:** Include herbal teas or supplements in your everyday regimen. Start with one or two and see how they impact your overall health.

**2. Listen to Your Body**: Observe how various herbs affect your body's reaction. To record your experiences and make any adjustments, keep a notebook.

**3. Establish a Morning Ritual**: Start the day with a few drops of a herbal tincture or a warm cup of herbal tea. This might establish an intention- and mindfulness-filled mood for the day.

**4. Use Herbs in Cooking:** Herbs provide health advantages in addition to flavor. Use them in cooking. Herbs that are fresh, such as rosemary, thyme, and basil, may improve both your meals and your health.

**5. Herbal Gardening:** Grow your own herbs if you have the room. This guarantees the quality of your treatments and links you to their source.

**6. Mindful Eating**: Pay attention to what you put in your body. When feasible, choose whole meals and organic foods to go along with your herbal medicines.

**7. Regular Movement**: Incorporate exercise into your herbal regimen. Exercise of any kind, including yoga and walking, promotes the body's natural distribution of the health benefits of herbs.

**8. Restorative Sleep**: To encourage a good night's sleep, which is crucial for general health, use relaxing herbs like lavender or chamomile.

**9. Stress Management**: Use adaptogenic herbs to strengthen the body's defenses against stress. Holy basil and ashwagandha are two herbs that might be used in a stress-reduction plan.

**10. Never Stop Learning**: Keep up with the latest information on holistic health and natural therapies. Read books, take part in workshops, and make connections with like-minded people.

Herbal medicines may be included into your everyday routine to help you maintain a healthy body, mind, and soul.

This section offers Beginners concrete strategies to use herbal treatments into their everyday life, making it both educational and useful. It is important to urge readers to get advice from healthcare professionals prior to beginning any new herbal regimen, particularly if they are using medication or have pre-existing health issues.

## Nutrition and Diet: The Foundation of Health

When it comes to using herbal home remedies, food and nutrition are the cornerstones that support actual health.

**1. Emphasize the Consumption of Whole** Foods—Fruits, Vegetables, Whole Grains, Nuts, and Seeds—Over Processed Foods: These foods provide vital nutrients and fiber.

**2. Balance is Key**: To guarantee a broad range of nutrients, a balanced diet consists of a variety of foods. The proportions of fats, proteins, and carbs in each meal should be balanced.

**3. Herbal Enhancements**: Add spices and herbs for flavor as well as their medicinal properties. Numerous plants provide important antioxidants, strengthen immunity, and facilitate digestion.

**4. Hydration**: Life requires water. Maintaining hydration facilitates the body's more efficient absorption of nutrients and herbal substances.

**5. Mindful Eating**: Savor your meal in the moment. Better digestion and a greater enjoyment of the food's inherent flavors are made possible by eating mindfully and slowly.

**6. Pay Attention to Your Body**: Your body communicates what it needs. Sometimes cravings are a sign of imbalances or shortages.

**7. Seasonal Eating:** Adapt your diet to the changing of the seasons. Foods that are in season tend to be higher in nutrients and more suited to the body's requirements.

**8. Moderation**: When consumed in excess, even the healthiest foods may be harmful. When it comes to anything, including herbal medications, exercise moderation.

**9. Individual demands**: Acknowledge that every person has different nutritional demands. One person's solution may not be another's.

**10. Never Stop Learning**: Keep up with the most recent findings in herbal medicine and nutrition. Having knowledge gives you the ability to choose what's best for your health.

You may build a solid foundation for health that supports the use of herbal treatments and a comprehensive approach to well-being by incorporating these ideas into your everyday life.

This part is designed to be both educational and user-friendly for novices, giving them the fundamental understanding needed to comprehend how nutrition, food, and herbal medicines interact. It's crucial to remind readers that dietary adjustments should be carefully considered and, if required, undertaken under the supervision of a healthcare provider.

# The Role of Exercise and Mindfulness

The Function of Physical Activity and Awareness in Herbal Home Treatments

For novices delving into the realm of herbal home medicines, comprehending the significance of exercise and mindfulness may significantly augment the path towards well-being.

1. **Exercise Boosts Efficacy**: Engaging in regular physical exercise may help the body better absorb and use herbal treatments. It increases circulation, which guarantees that the advantageous substances are dispersed efficiently.

2. **Mindfulness Enhances Healing**: Deep breathing exercises and other mindfulness techniques may augment the medicinal benefits of herbs. They aid in stress management, which is often the underlying cause of a number of health problems.

3. **Synergy with Yoga**: Herbal medicines may be very beneficial when used with yoga, which combines breath

and movement. Certain positions may facilitate relaxation, increase cleansing, and help with digestion.

**4. Nature as Therapy**: Nature, which is home to many medicinal plants, may be a soothing place to spend time. Exercise, awareness, and a closer relationship with the therapeutic qualities of plants are all made possible by it.

**5. Herbs to Promote Fitness**: Some herbs, such as turmeric, which has anti-inflammatory qualities, may promote fitness objectives and help the body recuperate from physical activity.

**6. Mindful Consumption**: Adding awareness to your meals will improve how well your body absorbs nutrients and herbal medicines, which will benefit your overall health.

**7. Stress-Relieving Herbs**: To successfully manage stress, combine mindfulness practices with herbs such as ashwagandha, lavender, and lemon balm.

**8. Consistent Practice:** Herbal treatments' effects may be enhanced and long-lasting health benefits can result from a daily exercise and mindfulness regimen.

**9. Tailored Approaches**: Just as herbal medicines should be customized to each patient's requirements and preferences, so too should mindfulness and fitness programmes.

**10. Learning and Adaptation**: As readers progress on their path to health, encourage them to seek out information on appropriate strategies and make adjustments to their routines.

Combining herbal treatments with exercise and mindfulness promotes a holistic approach to health that takes into account one's mental, emotional, and physical well-being.

# CONCLUSION

This book has served as a helpful introduction to the mild but potent realm of herbal medicine, which is a discipline that is as old as mankind itself and is still very much in use in our contemporary society.

This book has covered the fundamentals of herbal medicine, including the significance of appropriate dose and personalisation as well as sophisticated extraction methods. It has covered the skill of preservation, the morality of wildcrafting, and how to include these treatments into a holistic way of living that incorporates mindfulness, exercise, and proper diet.

Recall that achieving wellbeing is a personal and dynamic journey. Herbal medicines assist your body's natural healing processes while allowing you to harmonize with the cycles of the natural world. Have an open mind and a kind heart as you develop and learn more about herbal medicine. Remain interested, pay attention to your body, and show appreciation for the plants that provide us with their medicinal properties.

I hope you use this book as a reliable guide to harmony and wellness. Accept the knowledge of the herbs and allow them to lead you to a balanced, healthy existence.

I appreciate you getting this book to begin your herbal journey. I hope you have good health, joy, and a stronger connection with the natural world.

# Resources and Continuing Education

## Recommended Books and Websites

**Suggested Reading**
1.Lesley Bremness's book "The Complete Book of Herbs: A Practical Guide to Growing and Using Herbs"

**2.David Hoffmann's** book "Medical Herbalism: The Science and Practice of Herbal Medicine"

**3.James Green's** book "The Herbal Medicine-Maker's Handbook: A Home Manual"

**Websites for Additional Information**
**1."Encyclopedia** of Herbal Medicine" by Andrew Chevallier;

**2."Herbal Recipes** for Vibrant Health" by Rosemary Gladstar;

**Online classes are available at The Herbal** 1.Academy (herbalacademy.com), with levels ranging from basic to advanced.

2.The website Mountain Rose Herbs (mountainroseherbs.com) offers a wide range of herbal products, recipes, and information.

3.Leading authority in herbal education, the American Botanical Council (abc.herbalgram.org) provides materials and research.

4.United Plant Savers (united plant savers.org) provides educational tools and focuses on the protection of medicinal plants.

**Internet Communities and Forums**
1.**HerbMentor**: An online forum for all skill levels of herbalists (herbmentor.com).
(nimh.org.uk)

**2.The National** Institute of Medical Herbalists: provides materials and a database of licensed herbalists.

**Conferences and Workshops**
1.Global herbalists get together at the International Herb Symposium (internationalherbsymposium.com).

2.Herbal festivals and seminars in the area: Look for events on community boards and at nearby health food shops.

**Ongoing Education**
1.Take into consideration enrolling in classes in herbal medicine, holistic health, or botany at a nearby college or university.

2.Participate in seminars and workshops conducted by knowledgeable herbalists to get practical knowledge.

Rebecca Peters is a distinguished author in the fields of wellness and nutrition, whose passion for holistic health shines through her work. With a background enriched by diverse experiences in natural healing and dietary practices, Rebecca brings a wealth of knowledge to her readers.

Her commitment to wellness extends beyond her writing; Rebecca is a vocal advocate for sustainable living and the integration of natural remedies into everyday life. Her approach is characterized by a blend of traditional wisdom and contemporary nutritional science, making her insights both practical and forward-thinking.

Rebecca's book, "Herbal Home Remedy for Beginners," is a testament to her dedication to empowering others with the tools to improve their health naturally. Through her clear and accessible writing, she demystifies the world of herbal remedies, offering guidance that is both easy to understand and implement.

As an author, Rebecca's goal is to inspire her readers to embrace a more mindful approach to health, one that values the balance of body, mind, and spirit. Her work encourages a lifestyle that harmonizes with nature, advocating for the use of organic ingredients and the importance of listening to one's body.

Rebecca Peters continues to be a guiding light for those seeking to embark on a journey toward better health through natural means. Her contributions to the field of wellness and nutrition have made her a respected voice for those looking to lead a healthier, more holistic life.

www.ingramcontent.com/pod-product-compliance
Lightning Source LLC
Chambersburg PA
CBHW070805260726
48660CB00005B/1712